CONQUERING
Irritable Bowel Syndrome

A Guide to Liberating Those Suffering
with Chronic Stomach or Bowel Problems

D1531658

NICHOLAS J. TALLEY,
MD, PhD, MMedSci (Clin Epi), FRACP,
FRCP(Ed), FACP, FACG, FAFPHM

2006
BC Decker Inc
Hamilton

BC Decker Inc
P.O. Box 620, L.C.D. 1
Hamilton, Ontario L8N 3K7
Tel: 905-522-7017; 800-568-7281
Fax: 905-522-7839; 888-311-4987
E-mail: info@bcdecker.com
www.bcdecker.com

© 2006 BC Decker Inc

05 06 07/WPC/9 8 7 6 5 4 3 2 1

ISBN 1-896998-22-4
Printed in the United States
Cover image courtesy of the International Foundation for Functional Gastrointestinal Disorders.
Used with permission.

Sales and Distribution

United States
BC Decker Inc
P.O. Box 785
Lewiston, NY 14092-0785
Tel: 905-522-7017; 800-568-7281
Fax: 905-522-7839; 888-311-4987
E-mail: info@bcdecker.com
www.bcdecker.com

Canada
BC Decker Inc
20 Hughson Street South
P.O. Box 620, LCD 1
Hamilton, Ontario L8N 3K7
Tel: 905-522-7017; 800-568-7281
Fax: 905-522-7839; 888-311-4987
E-mail: info@bcdecker.com
www.bcdecker.com

Foreign Rights
John Scott & Company
International Publishers' Agency
P.O. Box 878
Kimberton, PA 19442
Tel: 610-827-1640
Fax: 610-827-1671
E-mail: jsco@voicenet.com

Japan
Igaku-Shoin Ltd.
Foreign Publications Department
3-24-17 Hongo
Bunkyo-ku, Tokyo, Japan 113-8719
Tel: 3 3817 5680
Fax: 3 3815 6776
E-mail: fd@igaku-shoin.co.jp

UK, Europe, Scandinavia, Middle East
Elsevier Science
Customer Service Department
Foots Cray High Street
Sidcup, Kent
DA14 5HP, UK
Tel: 44 (0) 208 308 5760
Fax: 44 (0) 181 308 5702
E-mail: cservice@harcourt.com

*Singapore, Malaysia, Thailand,
Philippines, Indonesia, Vietnam, Pacific
Rim, Korea*
Elsevier Science Asia
583 Orchard Road
#09/01, Forum
Singapore 238884
Tel: 65-737-3593
Fax: 65-753-2145

Australia, New Zealand
Elsevier Science Australia
Customer Service Department
STM Division
Locked Bag 16
St. Peters, New South Wales, 2044
Australia
Tel: 61 02 9517-8999
Fax: 61 02 9517-2249
E-mail: stmp@harcourt.com.au
www.harcourt.com.au

Mexico and Central America
ETM SA de CV
Calle de Tula 59
Colonia Condesa
06140 Mexico DF, Mexico
Tel: 52-5-5553-6657
Fax: 52-5-5211-8468
E-mail: editoresdetextosmex@
prodigy.net.mx

Brazil
Tecmedd Importadora E
Distribuidora De Livros Ltda.
Avenida Maurílio Biagi, 2850
City Ribeirão, Ribeirão Preto –
SP – Brasil
CEP: 14021-000
Tel: 0800 992236
Fax: (16) 3993-9000
E-mail: tecmedd@tecmedd.com.br

India, Bangladesh, Pakistan, Sri Lanka
Elsevier Health Sciences Division
Customer Service Department
17A/1, Main Ring Road
Lajpat Nagar IV
New Delhi – 110024, India
Tel: 91 11 2644 7160-64
Fax: 91 11 2644 7156
E-mail: esindia@vsnl.net

CONTENTS

ACKNOWLEDGMENTS

I would like to thank the many people who have helped me prepare this book. I am particularly grateful to Drs. Douglas Drossman, W. Grant Thompson, Lin Chang, Amit Sood, and Natasha Koloski, who provided expert input into various parts of this book.

I want to thank Dr. Sidney Phillips, now retired, for his mentorship and leadership in this field.

I must acknowledge all my family, and especially my sons, Nicholas and Mathew, for providing a reality check for me.

Finally, my students and patients have taught me so much and have made me realize there is still so much to learn; you are all an inspiration.

DEDICATION

This book is dedicated to my father, Dr. Nicholas Alexander Talley, a brilliant physician and true humanitarian and my grandfather Dr. Miklos Tallyai-Roth, an inspiration to us all.

"...it is impossible for me to describe adequately and truly in words the effects that IBS has had on my life. One of the reasons is that the effect is so major, and major things are difficult to talk about; another is that the symptoms (and their results) are so variable and interrelated, and that makes them difficult to describe; lastly, one wishes to be hopeful, positive, and optimistic, for one's sake and others, yet not underestimate the seriousness and distressfulness of the condition."

A Patient with IBS

Cramps or pain in the stomach; feelings of bloating or even of swelling up like a balloon; having to rush to the toilet because of diarrhea, or not being able to go at all—these are some of the symptoms of irritable bowel syndrome (IBS). Up to 1 in 10 Americans are troubled by typical IBS symptoms, and most have not seen a doctor about them. In some cases the complaints are minor; in others, IBS unfortunately rules the person's life. IBS costs taxpayers billions of dollars each year because of medication use and consultations with doctors or alternative therapists.

Many doctors know little about IBS, and many dismiss patients' IBS symptoms as being "in their heads." Huge numbers of people suffer with IBS, yet treatment is often ineffective or works only for a while before its effect wears off. Diets, often tried, can make symptoms worse for some. Other sufferers are advised to self-medicate when the symptoms are worse, but how best to do this? New drugs claimed to be helpful have hit the market very recently, but are they safe and effective? Many people seek alternative care, but is this approach always safe? And does it work?

Thankfully, a quiet revolution that looks as if it will help is going on. First, ways of evaluating whether treatments really work (so-called evidence-based medicine) are being applied to IBS with surprising results. Second, alternative therapies are going under the scientific microscope, and indeed, some do seem to be useful although others seem useless. Third, new medications have finally arrived and can help. Finally, there are intriguing hints that IBS has a cause and that a cure may eventually be within our reach.

Knowledge is power. Those who are troubled with IBS need to take control by understanding the problem and potential solutions. This book aims to help empower IBS sufferers and their families. It covers what IBS is, why some people may get the disease, and what measures that really work can be taken now.

I am very grateful to all the patients who have taught me so much about the problem and the struggle to manage it.

I thank the Mayo Clinic Medical Education Department for granting me permission to use some of the excellent patient education materials included in this book.

I thank the men and women who have written to me about their IBS and have allowed me to quote their words; all of you have inspired me to write about this human condition and its consequences.

Nicholas J. Talley
August 2005

As the founder of a nonprofit organization dedicated to providing assistance to individuals with gastrointestinal disorders, I know firsthand the frustrations individuals with irritable bowel syndrome (IBS) experience in trying to make sense of their disorder. If you are one of those individuals, I invite you into this book. *Conquering Irritable Bowel Syndrome* provides a comprehensive overview of IBS. This is a book that speaks to the individual who lives with, copes with, and struggles to manage the symptoms of IBS.

I first met Dr. Nick Talley more than a decade ago, when my own involvement in the medical community and the world of gastroenterology was just beginning. When I started the International Foundation for Functional Gastrointestinal Disorders, there were few gastroenterologists devoting their careers to research in IBS and to the clinical care of patients with IBS; Nick was one of them. Nick continues to be a driving force in the field. His involvement is far-reaching, ranging from the study of genes that may contribute to IBS to explorations into the treatment of IBS with Chinese herbal medicine.

IBS is a chronic disorder for which there is no cure and few treatments that address its numerous symptoms. Patients often get caught in an unending search for medications or for any remedy that can provide relief of their symptoms. Drug development, clinical trials, and how a drug is determined to be safe and effective are particularly important to those living with a chronic illness. Much needed insight into these processes is found in Chapter 4, "Taking Control: What Treatments Really Work?" This chapter points out the importance of evidence-based decisions when treatment is being chosen and provides guidance to help patients (and their physicians) determine what may work best for them. There is also a discussion about the placebo effect, which I think everyone who has IBS needs to be aware of.

The search for relief can take IBS sufferers in many different directions, some confusing and others unproductive. This book addresses many of the questions often asked by those who are diagnosed with IBS as well as by those who are wondering if they have the disease.

You may see a story in this book that you recognize as your own and may realize that you are not alone. Millions of people live every day with the symptoms of IBS. While the level of severity varies, the fact remains that the symptoms of IBS can and do have an impact on quality of life. For many people, that means having to continually make adjustments in their lives, often diminishing their personal or professional potential.

Conquering Irritable Bowel Syndrome describes how our definition of IBS has evolved "from a broad all-encompassing intestinal condition to what is now a more specific concept." It is the more specific nature of IBS that is being defined now, and this enables scientists to move closer to finding answers and valuable solutions for patients.

We are moving forward in our efforts to conquer IBS. Nick's sensitive and insightful presentation in these pages adds important and useful information to the knowledge base from which patients can draw. Thus armed with a clearer understanding, individuals with IBS can make more informed choices in their efforts to effectively manage its individualized symptoms.

Nancy Norton

CHAPTER 1

WHAT IS IRRITABLE BOWEL SYNDROME?

"I have had IBS spastic colon since I was 10, 57 years ago."

"I could write a book, myself, about what I went through with IBS, but I'm on the other end of my life, being 81 years old."

"My life is happy and stress free, except for the fact that I suffer daily from IBS."

Maybe you wake up in the morning feeling fine, but a few minutes later, you start to feel a gnawing discomfort or pain in your lower stomach. There may be waves of discomfort followed by relief, or the discomfort may be constant. When you go to the toilet and empty your bowels, the discomfort or pain is relieved but only temporarily. You may feel a sudden urge to run to the toilet, or you may try to go more frequently because you feel "plugged up." You may need to strain excessively but may be able to pass only very hard small stool if anything. On the other hand, you have very loose and frequent stool, or the pattern may change without your knowing why. You might notice a white slimy material (mucus) on the stool. Maybe you notice that your stomach feels full of gas and sometimes even swells up as if you were pregnant. If you have these types of symptoms, you could be suffering from irritable bowel syndrome. The following are a few illustrative examples of people suffering from this condition.

- *First-Date Diarrhea.* Sarah is an attractive 19-year-old woman who met Carl in college. She remembers having to find a bathroom every place they went during their first date. She was nervous and ended up opening her bowels, which helped relieve her cramping abdominal pain. Even more embarrassing, she would stain her underpants with a small amount of brown liquid stool. Drinking alcohol sometimes made the whole problem worse. She and Carl have fallen in love, but she is terrified of any intimacy because of embarrassment about her problem.

- *Gassing the Train.* Simone is 51 years old and is particularly worried about her problem with gas. She experiences abdominal pain and swelling, at times associated with either constipation or diarrhea. In addition, she noisily passes excess gas from her bowel at the most inappropriate times. She works for a large company and is still hoping to go up the business ladder but is terrified that she will pass gas in meetings and that this will be either heard or smelled by everyone. Upon catching the train, particularly in the morning, she would feel an urgent need (associated with passing gas) to go to the toilet and would have to step off the train and find a restroom.

- *Pseudopregnant.* Susan is a 38-year-old mother of two children who complains bitterly about abdominal swelling. When she gets up in the morning, her abdomen is flat, but it begins to swell soon after lunch. This can take some hours to settle and happens irregularly. She often feels that her abdominal discomfort is lessened when she has a bowel movement, and she also experiences some constipation. She feels incompletely empty after passing stool, as if she had not properly delivered the contents. Sometimes she sees some white slimy material on her stool. The main problem, though, remains the swelling. She has shown her husband, who is amazed. When she goes out shopping despite the swelling, she sometimes feels that people look at her oddly. She struggles to maintain a normal lifestyle.

- *The Squirter.* Peter is a 48-year-old high-flying executive under considerable stress at work as his company shares plummet and pressure mounts for the business to outperform its competitors. Peter describes terrible urgency. He has to race to the bathroom as soon as he feels the need to go. If he is not near a bathroom, he will leak liquid stool into his underpants. He often needs to spend 20 minutes several times in the morning sitting on the toilet and trying to clear his bowels before he drives to work. For this reason, he gets up even earlier than needed to prepare for work. On the drive in to work, he has to stop somewhere to empty his bowels. Peter knows every restroom between home and work on his commute. He never is constipated but often has diarrhea with pain that is relieved when he starts to pass the stool. He often feels a bit nauseated but never vomits. His symptoms are interfering with his work, and his wife feels most unhappy because of Peter's mood swings. Peter believes that his bowels are the main reason for the mood swings but doesn't know what to do about the problem.

- *The Strainer.* Heather is a 24-year-old model. She is thin and fit, but her lifestyle is disturbed by bowel dysfunction. Heather has to strain excessively to have a bowel movement. She has a bowel movement only once or twice per week. She sometimes notices a white slimy material on the stool, and she often feels incompletely empty after going, but she never has diarrhea. Heather does not eat a lot and wants to stay thin for her modeling profession. She usually has abdominal discomfort until she goes to the toilet to empty her bowels, and she often feels bloated although her abdomen never visibly swells up. She also often feels nauseated. Her diet is irregular. She is very afraid she might have a serious disease.

IRRITABLE BOWEL SYNDROME: WHAT IS IT?

Irritable bowel syndrome (IBS) remains a relatively mysterious and often hidden problem. Until recently, it was not appreciated that IBS affects at least 1 in 10 Americans. Professor Grant

Thompson (a Canadian) and Ken Heaten (from England) were among the first to bring attention to the prevalence of IBS when they published their report of a large survey of 301 volunteers from England in 1980. It seemed amazing how common bowel symptoms were in people otherwise considered healthy, and most sufferers had not consulted a doctor for the problem.[1] My work at the Mayo Clinic has only served to confirm these findings.[2,3] More than 10% of otherwise healthy persons in the United States have IBS-like symptoms, and many more have constipation or diarrhea, with no stomach pain. Older terms that were used to describe IBS include spastic colitis and mucous colitis ("colitis" means inflammation in the colon), but as obvious inflammation is absent in IBS, these terms have not been in vogue for many years.

Over time, the definition of IBS has evolved from a broad all-encompassing intestinal condition to what is now a more specific concept. Complaints about stomach or bowel problems are remarkably common in the community. Table 1-1 lists gastrointestinal disorders and the percentage of the population affected by each disorder. It is striking that only about one-third of the population has absolutely no stomach or bowel complaints; this means that it is abnormal to have no abdominal symptoms at all! However, not everyone with stomach or bowel symptoms has IBS. We now recognize that IBS is just one of a large group of unexplained chronic intestinal problems. This means that although the symptoms are real, there is no obvious change in the structure of the bowel to explain them. Rather, it seems that in many cases, these symptoms may be due to enhanced sensitivity of the bowel, often associated with abnormalities in the way the bowel moves the material within it (a concept discussed later in this book).

Follow-up studies indicate that the proportion of the population that is suffering with these symptoms appears to be

Table 1-1: Functional Gastrointestinal Disorders (Rome Classification) and Their Frequency in the United States

Disorder	People Affected in the United States (%)
Functional esophageal disorders	
Globus (feeling of a lump in the throat)	1
Chest pain	5
Heartburn (once a week or more)	20
Trouble swallowing	5
Functional gastroduodenal disorders	
Functional (nonulcer) dyspepsia	15–20
Air swallowing	3
Vomiting	< 1
Functional bowel disorders	
Irritable bowel syndrome (IBS)	10–15
Bloating	4
Constipation	3
Diarrhea	2
Abdominal pain (not from IBS)	1
Gallbladder pain	< 1
Functional anorectal disorders	
Leakage of stool (incontinence)	2
Pain (anal)	8

remarkably constant from year to year. However, some people lose their symptoms over time while other people are developing these symptoms for the first time. The two groups balance each other, which accounts for the stability of the rate of the condition each year. It is interesting that some bowel symptoms decline as the person ages (Figure 1-1). However, IBS and other gastrointestinal complaints remain common in elderly people and are often misdiagnosed as being due to other causes, such as pockets (bulges) in the large bowel (a condition called diverticulosis).

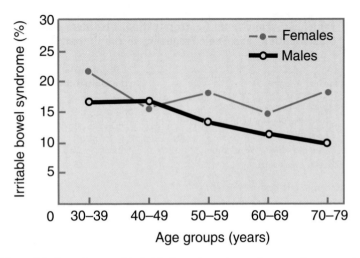

Figure 1-1: Prevalence of irritable bowel syndrome in a random sample of a representative county (Olmsted County, MN) in the United States (n = 1,163). Reproduced with permission from Talley NJ. Functional gastrointestinal disorders. In: Friedman SL, McQuaid KR, Grendell JH, editors. Current diagnosis and treatment in gastroenterology. 2nd ed. McGraw-Hill; 2003.

SYMPTOMS OF IRRITABLE BOWEL SYNDROME

The patient with IBS complains about discomfort or pain in the abdomen. However, this pain is also linked to diarrhea, constipation, or both diarrhea and constipation; the combination of symptoms is key to making the diagnosis correctly. Let's consider the following complaints of some patients with documented IBS:

- "I was first diagnosed with IBS 20 years ago. I had just had my first child, and I had to leave her to go to work. I cried and cried every day. Needless to say, I ended up with terrible stomach cramps, bloating, gas, and diarrhea and constipation."

- "Everywhere I went I had to know where the bathroom was—how far I was from the bathroom."
- "No one day is the same. I might have diarrhea, and then I'll be constipated."
- "I am a 68-year-old retired university physics professor. I have had severe IBS attacks continually for 35 years. All the medical tests have shown that nothing else is causing my extreme discomfort, other than IBS. My symptoms are nausea, bloating, urgency, and pain."

Note that these people complain of abdominal discomfort or pain. If questioned closely, many will say the discomfort or pain is made better when they empty their bowels. Alternatively, the onset of the pain or discomfort is directly linked to either an increase or a decrease in the frequency of bowel movements, or to a change in the looseness or hardness of the stool. It is this close association between abdominal pain or discomfort and change in bowel function that defines IBS according to current international diagnostic criteria (the Rome criteria).

IBS can be conceived as a condition causing the "ABCs." What is meant by this? Basically, IBS is characterized by the following:

- **A**bdominal (stomach) pain or discomfort
- **B**loating or visible swelling (as if pregnant)
- **C**onstipation
- **D**iarrhea
- **E**xtra bowel symptoms in some cases (such as tiredness, headaches, backaches, or muscle aches)

Diarrhea (from Greek, meaning "to flow") in IBS typically manifests as loose or watery stools. There is usually no blood seen. Constipation (from the Latin *constipatio*, meaning "to crowd together") can mean hard stools or infrequent bowel movements. Sometimes, people strain a lot or squeeze around the anus or vagina to help pass stool. Some people with IBS alternate between diarrhea and constipation, with their abdominal pain or discomfort.

It is very important to recognize that in a number of people, IBS is not confined to just stomach or bowel symptoms. This implies, at least for such persons, that there is some kind of generalized abnormality of body function that can lead to the problem. What are some of these common extra bowel symptoms? It has been shown that many people with IBS feel tired or fatigued. The trouble is, being tired is very common in this modern world, and stress certainly plays a role in causing such feelings. However, people with IBS tend to be more fatigued than others, at least in a subset. Back pain is also more common, as are pains around the muscles and joints (which may lead to a diagnosis of fibromyalgia). Urinary symptoms (including feelings of urgency and having to go to the toilet more frequently) are more common in IBS. This suggests that not only is the bowel irritable in some people but that the bladder is also irritable. Indeed, the muscle in the wall of the bladder and the muscle in the bowel (both of which are of a type called *smooth muscle*) are remarkably similar in many ways, which could explain this association. Migraine headaches are more common in people with IBS than in people without this problem. Even asthma, which is due to hyperreactivity of the bronchial smooth muscle in the airways, seems to be more common in people with IBS.

So, it is important to realize that if you have other symptoms besides your intestinal symptoms, all of them could be caused by the one disease process. Certainly, it is important to talk about all of your symptoms with your physician in order to avoid unnecessary tests or surgeries being performed because of your other symptoms. Unfortunately, a woman with IBS is more likely to lose her uterus, or any individual his or her gallbladder, because of having presented with abdominal pain that was not correctly diagnosed at the time. Indeed, it can be very difficult to work out the exact cause of pain at the beginning; doctors and patients may not recognize the presence of IBS symptoms that could explain the problem. The diagnosis of IBS may just not be considered by any party in the heat of the moment.

We do not know exactly why IBS can present with all of these extra intestinal manifestations, but (as will be discussed later) the fact that the brain's processing of pain signals from the body can be abnormal in IBS could be one key factor.

Many people, however, will not have the full set of features of IBS. For example, they may have only abdominal pain or discomfort, with relatively normal bowel function. On the other hand, their bowel function may be abnormal, with diarrhea, constipation, or alternating diarrhea and constipation, yet abdominal pain or discomfort may be either absent or only a minor component. Currently, people in these groups are not classified as having IBS but usually have what is called a *functional gastrointestinal disorder* (this term is a mouthful, I know). "Functional" is a term commonly used in the medical literature and on the Internet and therefore is included here. It means that there is no obvious structural explanation for the gastrointestinal complaints; thus, the inside of the bowel seems quite normal, even if its functioning (the way it moves its contents along) is not normal. In the past, "functional" also had other meanings, including (regrettably) the implication that the symptoms are due to some type of psychiatric disease or psychological process. However, in current usage, the word carries no implication that the symptoms are from any particular cause; it means only that there is no definite structural explanation for them.

In the old days, "functional" was often used interchangeably with "hysteria." Many doctors still think this way although attitudes are changing. "If you cannot find a cause, surely it's only in their heads" has held sway for too long in the medical world. In the days before syphilis was recognized as an infectious disease, for example, some of its manifestations were attributed to psychiatric disturbance! Certainly, in the first 85 years of the twentieth century, peptic ulcer disease was usually attributed to a psychosomatic or psychological condition. Peptic ulcers are deep holes in the lining of the stomach (or in the upper small bowel) caused by acid damage. Indeed, the fact that stomach acid secretion does increase with stress lent further support to the concept that peptic ulcers must have a strong psychological component. However, it is now clear that all of this thinking was completely wrong. Barry Marshall, a young Australian physician-in-training who was working on a research project with Dr. Robin Warren, observed that loads of bacteria were present in stomach biopsy specimens from most people with stomach ulcers (Figure 1-2).[4] We now know that peptic ulcers are primarily due either to this infectious agent (*Helicobacter pylori*) (see Figure 1-2) or to aspirin or other antiarthritis drugs (called nonsteroidal antiinflammatory drugs). Since the discovery of the infectious cause of peptic ulcers (which was confirmed when it was found that the elimination of the bacteria healed the ulcers and prevented relapse), the interest in psychological factors in ulcer disease has essentially disappeared (as it should have). For their discovery, Dr. Marshall and Dr. Warren have been nominated for the Nobel Prize.

A complete list of functional gastrointestinal disorders is presented in Appendix 1. Note that the symptoms of these disorders vary but have the common characteristic of being currently unexplained yet common problems. Of course, some of these symptoms can also be due to other conditions. For example, heartburn is a burning sensation in the chest or stomach that rises up toward the throat, most often because of

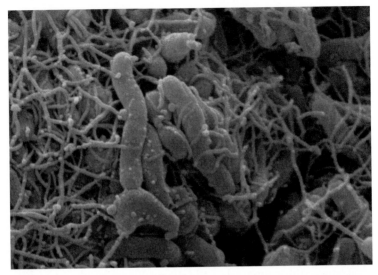

Figure 1-2: Numerous bacteria (*Helicobacter pylori*) live on the surface lining of the stomach and cause stomach inflammation that can lead to peptic ulcers (but not to irritable bowel syndrome). Photo compliments of Dr. H. H. Xia, University of Hong Kong.

acid reflux into the esophagus. Acid in the esophagus can cause damage (called esophagitis) although this does not occur in everybody; indeed, most people with excessive acid reflux have no esophageal damage. Studies have shown, however, that some people who experience typical heartburn do not have excessive acid in the esophagus; this condition is called functional heartburn.

Another very common condition is pain or discomfort in the upper stomach area, which is above the navel (the belly button) but below the chest. This is called *dyspepsia* in the medical literature (from Greek, literally meaning "bad digestion") although this term is not used by most people outside of the medical profession. Pain or discomfort in the upper stomach area can occasionally be due to a peptic ulcer and very rarely to a stomach cancer, but there is most frequently no evidence of an ulcer or any other obvious cause. Doctors label such persons as having *nonulcer dyspepsia* because there is no obvious explanation (such as an ulcer) for the symptoms. In recent years, a more popular term for nonulcer dyspepsia has been *functional dyspepsia* because it is assumed that a disorder of stomach function contributes to causing the symptoms. About one-third of people with IBS also complain of upper stomach discomfort or pain and also have functional dyspepsia.

MY PERSONAL SEARCH TO UNDERSTAND
IRRITABLE BOWEL SYNDROME

How and why did I develop an interest in IBS? To understand this, you need to know a little about me and about my background, so I will relay this tale to you.

I am a third-generation physician. I became fascinated by the mind-body relationship in school and followed up on this passion in my research after medical school. My father, also a gastroenterologist, was born in Hungary but did his medical training in Sydney, Australia. His father was a chest physician in Budapest and was well known for his expertise in tuberculosis. Dr. Miklos Tallyai-Roth (my father's name was Tallyai, at his father's insistence) worked at the Koranyi Clinik (1906-1923) and rose to be Adjunct (head, under Prof. Baron Sandor Koranyi, my father's godfather); he then became director of the Erzsebet-Weiss Manfred Sanatorium for Lung Diseases (now the Hungarian Institute of Pulmonology at Budakeszi). He was invited to take up a professorial position in the United States not long before World War II but sadly turned it down. My father had a privileged background. However, he lost his mother when he was 4 years old; as a result, he was brought up by his father and a nanny who spoke English, which became the preferred language in the home. The war brought disaster, though; the Nazis arrested my father and grandfather, and my grandfather died a week later under very mysterious circumstances. My father was released only to go through the usual and well-known tribulations that affected people in Hungary under first the German and then the Russian occupation. Ultimately, he ended up in a Russian prisoner-of-war camp but luckily escaped while accompanying some sick prisoners to a local hospital (he had told the Russians that as a medical student, he was so qualified). He had to hide out in a haystack that was bayoneted by pursuing soldiers, but he did escape. From there, he was later able to return to Budapest and take one room in the old apartment that he had previously owned and which was now occupied by multiple families. By August 1945, he was able to sit and pass the university exams in medicine for the first and second years (the university was closed in March 1944, but he had done most of the required 2 years of work), but the political climate became blacker and blacker. Following the collapse of the Nazi occupation, the country was inexorably becoming a communist Russian satellite, and he started looking for an opportunity to escape to the West. He was actually advised to choose between joining the Communist Party or getting out by the new professor of medicine, who had been installed by the communist powers but who was also an old friend of his father. He was fortunate enough to get papers for a short trip to Prague and decided to flee; he then went to the United States consulate in Prague. My father found a kind US official who was so amazed by his English that he granted a temporary visa to the US for my father. And so Dad caught a plane and arrived in New York. There he decided to move on to Sydney, Australia, because he had a cousin living "down under" and because the Australian government had issued him an entry permit. Dad arrived penniless but then put himself through medical school in Sydney (the Hungarian exam scores were not accepted), working nights (often all night) and going to the university during the day. He was fortunate enough to receive a scholarship in his third year. He changed his surname to Talley to avoid the negativity directed at migrants in Australia in those days.

I was born in Perth, Australia. Perth used to be a sleepy town with a reputation (still held to this day) for being the city furthest from any other major city in the world. It is a place full of independent-minded individuals. My father was a medical resident undertaking pediatric training for a year. When I was 6 months old, however, we moved back to Sydney so that my father could pursue training in adult medicine at the most prestigious training hospital in the country, Royal Prince Alfred Hospital. Dad became a gastroenterologist (ie, an abdominal specialist and one of the early pioneers in the country) and has had a very distinguished career in clinical medicine in Sydney.

I was educated in a Jesuit Catholic school (St. Aloysius College). The Jesuits taught critical thinking and emphasized the acquisition of rational evidence-based opinions; I greatly benefited from their sharp minds and their philosophic perspective. The school's environment instilled a passion for seeking the truth and for considering the evidence; the teachers wanted each pupil to reach his or her full potential, and I believe they did a good job therein with my peers.

The biggest turning point in my life, though, was at the age of 10 years and not in Australia but in the United States. At that time, my father was awarded a research fellowship to go to Chicago and work with Dr. Joseph Kirshner, a famous researcher in inflammatory bowel disease. We arrived in Chicago in late November in the midst of a very cold winter (my first with snow), and I enrolled in the nearby public school. For some inexplicable reason, I was enormously stimulated by this change. One teacher told my shocked parents that I must be a "genius" because I liked to read so much (my parents had to this point despaired of my making it to college, ever). My parents noted a dramatic difference in terms of my academic focus, which had been almost nonexistent prior to our moving. I left the United States, absolutely determined to succeed academically, which I realized could occur only through very hard work. This has held me in good stead ever since. I went to medical school at the University of New South Wales in Sydney. The medical curriculum at the time I began university was undergoing radical change, and I was in the first year of a trial 5-year medical degree program that did not last. My time at the university, however, remains one of the most joyous memories I have; I thrived in an environment of hard work, scientific thought, and humanistic interest. Ever since, I have been a passionate advocate for the art of medicine as well as its science.

My undergraduate medical training was at the St. George Hospital in Sydney, where my father was on the staff. During this time, I came under the influence of Prof. Robert Pitney, a distinguished hematologist (blood specialist) who taught me how to listen to and examine patients. His influence, among that of others, stimulated me to later write a series of books on clinical methods, books still widely used in medical schools around the world. Toward the end of my medical course, I became interested in research, but I did not undertake any formal research training at the time because of my desire to graduate and to practice medicine; I was eager to help others and thought I knew so much (and how wrong can one be?). After graduation, I undertook my internship and residency at the Prince of Wales Hospital in Sydney, arguably still the leading teaching hospital of the University of New South Wales. After physician basic training at the Prince of Wales Hospital for 2 years, I was at a bit of a loss. I wanted to do research, but I still needed to complete my training. I looked around at options and discussed all of this with my father, who gave me the first of two pieces of superb advice that would change my life: He suggested I consider a research scholarship at Royal North Shore Hospital that was being offered by Prof. Douglas Piper. I really wasn't sure I wanted to become a gastroenterologist (the brain seemed much more interesting), but I decided to explore the possibility.

Prof. Piper (Doug) was a particularly distinguished investigator in peptic ulcer disease. He was very bright and full of ideas, and the medical students loved him as a teacher because he simplified everything brilliantly. However, when he lectured, he sometimes tended to mumble in his rather broad Australian accent, and some (especially those who were not Australian) had real difficulty following what he was saying. Doug had a small team of dedicated nurses working with him but no full-time PhD students when I expressed an interest in coming. At the time, clinical research into conditions such as IBS or peptic ulcer was looked down upon as being of minor importance; only those who were studying cells or other basic mechanisms of disease were considered to be doing important work. We spoke, and Doug initially wanted me to study ulcer disease; I decided to "take a punt" and work with him. Luckily, the first grant we requested, for research on the natural history of peptic ulcers, was not awarded, so we decided to look at another topic that fascinated me. In many of our patients who had ulcer symptoms (such as bad indigestion with stomach pain), no ulcer crater or ulcer scar could be found when we looked down into the stomach with an endoscope (a type of camera). And this seemed to be common although we had no idea how common. This entity had a new name, nonulcer dyspepsia, but was totally mysterious. I realized that some of the pain being reported could be due to IBS or acid reflux in some cases, but the pain was not caused by either of these in other cases, and I wanted to understand it. I then spent 3 years at Royal North Shore Hospital undertaking research into nonulcer dyspepsia that led to the award of a PhD degree. We learned much: nonulcer dyspepsia was much more common than peptic ulcer; about a third of patients with nonulcer dyspepsia had IBS; acid suppression therapy was of minimal benefit; gastric emptying was slow in some cases; stress was not a big factor; and symptoms persisted in the long term, yet few developed ulcer disease.

I loved research and the research environment at Royal North Shore Hospital, and I have continued to pursue research passionately ever since. I also found I was drawn to the study of the bowel diseases we knew so little about. I asked myself, what is nonulcer dyspepsia, and why is it related to IBS? Is it the same condition just presenting differently? Why were some of the patients in my studies so incapacitated by their symptoms even though there was no medical explanation for their complaints? Was this a mental problem or a physical problem, or both, or neither? Could it be cured?

I would spend a further year doing gastroenterologic clinical and research work at Royal North Shore Hospital before traveling to the United States to take up a research fellowship with Prof. Sydney Phillips at the Mayo Clinic in Rochester, MN. This was yet another chance event! I had written to a number of distinguished institutions in North America, inquiring about prospective research positions as I wished to follow up on my work on nonulcer dyspepsia. I had planned to go to one of the centers doing ulcer research, but here my father gave me the second piece of advice that would change my destiny. He told me I must write to Dr. Sidney (Sid) Phillips at the Mayo Clinic. Sid was known to my dad because he was an Australian, originally from Melbourne. So I wrote to him, but only as an afterthought. I finally chose the Mayo Clinic because it was the first institution to offer me a paid fellowship, which was enormously attractive at that point in my career. This was very fortunate; taking up the Mayo Clinic research fellowship was one of the best career decisions I have ever made.

I spent 18 months in the Gastroenterology Research Unit with Sid, undertaking new research. For the first time, I was exposed to an environment in which world authorities were conducting cutting-edge clinical and basic research; I was enormously stimulated by the brilliant people around me. When I was offered a position on the staff, I shelved my plans to travel to Canada and Europe for further experience and spent another 5½ years at the Mayo Clinic. I might well have stayed longer, but by chance, I met the wife of the new Associate Dean of the Western Clinical School at the University of Sydney at a conference in Minneapolis. I was asked if I might be interested in applying for a foundation Chair of Medicine at a new small teaching hospital, the Nepean Hospital in the west of Sydney. I elected to apply after much soul searching and was successful. I subsequently spent 9 years at the Nepean Hospital, undertaking research, teaching, practicing gastroenterology, and building (as chief) a new Division of Medicine. In 2002, I returned to the Mayo Clinic after being made a wonderful offer to undertake research work. I am currently a professor of medicine in the Mayo Clinic College of Medicine and am pursuing my passions, namely, research, teaching, and patient care.

My research continues to focus on the unexplained functional gastrointestinal disorders. I am intrigued by the accumulated evidence that the functional gastrointestinal disorders can aggregate in families, and the work we have undertaken with twins consistently suggests the existence of a genetic contribution. We are actively pursuing the hypothesis that the functional gastrointestinal disorders are genetically based, at least in part, and I am convinced that this effort will lead to substantial progress in terms of new diagnostic tests and treatments. We are continuing also to study what happens to the functional gastrointestinal disorders over time and the role of environmental factors that may interact with genes. We are evaluating what goes wrong in the bowel and how we can fix it with drugs or machines. We want to find the causes and cures!

HIGH COST OF IRRITABLE BOWEL SYNDROME: PATIENTS' REFLECTIONS

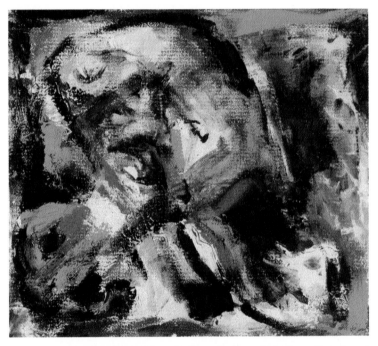

Pain, from the International Foundation for the Functional Gastrointestinal Disorders (IFFGD) Art of IBS Collection. Printed with permission from the IFFGD (©2004 IFFGD).

"My life has been extremely affected by IBS. I first got signs of IBS when I was 15, and I was diagnosed at 16. I'm 18, almost 19 now, and I'm really happy to hear that there are so many other people out there like me. I like to eat. I get really angry sometimes when I want to eat something, and I know I shouldn't have it because it will upset

my stomach. IBS caused me to miss numerous days of school to where I almost got in trouble for truancy. All the days I missed at school caused me to fall behind on my work; so I couldn't catch up, and I failed that semester, when I was used to getting A's and B's."

"IBS wears the experiencer down so much, physically and otherwise, that one can well imagine it making one more vulnerable and susceptible to other damaging conditions, which might be life threatening."

"This condition makes it difficult to function, and I fear leaving the house or leaving a place with an available bathroom. It has affected my relationships, especially my marriage and my friendships, as I feel misunderstood, and I often burden others with my complaints. Others are always worried about asking how poor K feels, and though I appreciate the concern, I hate being that person who everyone worries about or, if someone else is driving, has to rush to a bathroom."

"I fear an IBS attack. There is the ever-present lack of predictability in your life, and this causes lots of stress."

"I have had a heart attack and lots of routine operations and have had chronic migraine ("aura") headaches. However, none of these have come anywhere near to causing the stress in my life as the chronic IBS attack."

"I have experienced so much frustration, embarrassment, and anger over this condition and have felt miserably misunderstood and dismissed."

"After eating, more often than not I have to rush to a bathroom with diarrhea, usually about 20 minutes after a meal. Usually, it will occur several times. Finding a bathroom becomes an urgent, stressful experience, wherever I go. The pain I experience on a daily basis is so bad that I am routinely doubled over and have to lie down. My IBS rules my life. It is relentless and does not subside."

"Sometimes it wakes me out of sound sleep, and sometimes you could be standing talking to someone and you do not have time to react. It is explosive diarrhea, and you have no control over it. It has proved to be quite humiliating at times."

"I am a 68-year-old retired university physics professor. I have tried all the pertinent drugs for IBS and have had extensive psychotherapy. Nothing has helped quell the terrible problems associated with IBS. My wife is a real savior during these attacks. I have even contemplated suicide but never came close to acting on this impulse. When the IBS attack is over or at least tolerable, my mental attitude becomes very good again. Severe IBS is a horrendous disease to live with. It robs you of your ability to look forward to future events (in the short and long term)."

I know from my patients that IBS varies from very mild to very severe. The condition can destroy some people's quality of life. The costs to the community are enormous—in the billions of dollars annually, at least, for tests and treatments.[5] I also know that IBS can be a chronic condition and can be very stressful. This book has been written to help people manage this problem. "Knowledge is power," said Sir Francis Bacon in 1597, and this book aims to empower you so that relief or at least some sense of control can be gained.

Take-Home Messages

- IBS is common; if you have the disease, you are not alone!
- IBS causes abdominal discomfort or pain that typically comes and goes.
- IBS causes diarrhea, constipation, or alternating diarrhea and constipation.
- IBS often causes bloating; in some people, the abdomen may visibly swell up.
- IBS symptoms are typically unpredictable.
- IBS can vary from a minor annoyance to an incapacitating problem.
- IBS is a real disease.

CHAPTER 2

HOW COMMON IS IRRITABLE BOWEL SYNDROME, AND HOW IS IT DIAGNOSED?

"You can observe a lot by watching." (Yogi Berra, 1925)

HOW COMMON IS THE PROBLEM, OR AM I ALONE?

"The most important thing for experiencers of IBS (a better word than "sufferers") is to know that they are not alone. Many others are experiencing whatever they are experiencing. Fellow experiencers can help one another by mutual moral and pragmatic support. We need more support groups, one in each community."

You are definitely not alone if you suffer with irritable bowel syndrome (IBS) or a related condition; of 290 million Americans in 2005, a staggering 29 million (10% of the population) have IBS. Furthermore, two-thirds of the population experience some stomach or bowel symptoms that come and go. Indeed, if you do not suffer with any gastrointestinal complaints ever, you are probably a little abnormal (but lucky!).[1] The good news is that IBS never kills you and does not predispose you to cancer or inflammatory bowel disease. But some of the tests and treatments can cause harm, and you'll learn about those issues in this book.

Only a small number of people go to their doctor and complain about their stomach or bowel symptoms. From community surveys in the United States and all around the world, we know that only about 1 in 4 people with IBS seek traditional medical care. Some others seek out alternative practitioners to help them. Others just use over-the-counter medications. Still others just put up with their symptoms or may be able to control them with simple diet changes or other approaches that are described in detail later in this book.

What drives people to seek medical care? This remains remarkably mysterious. We know that people who have more severe symptoms certainly are more likely to go to their doctor. This is just common sense but has been confirmed in numerous studies. However, symptom severity seems to be only a minor factor in driving people to see physicians, which is surprising. Other studies suggest that those people who are particularly concerned that they may have some kind of really serious health problem will seek care (fear of cancer is particularly common). Other people actually may be afraid to seek care, fearing that a serious health problem may be found. People under stress or people who are particularly anxious or even depressed seem to be more likely to see a doctor about their bowel problems. The association between stress and bowel

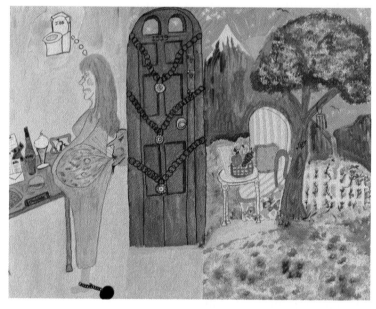

Untitled, from the International Foundation for Functional Gastrointestinal Disorders (IFFGD) Art of IBS Collection. Printed with permission from the IFFGD (©2004 IFFGD).

problems is covered in detail later on, but it is clear that there is a link, at least in some cases, and addressing both the bowel problems and the stress can be helpful. However, this does not apply to everybody, by any means.

Women tend to see doctors more than do men about these kinds of complaints although this may not be so in all parts of the world. For example, in India, more men than women present with IBS, and this has been attributed to cultural factors: in the West, it is more socially acceptable for women to go to doctors than for men to do so whereas the opposite is the case in India. Your behavior in terms of deciding to see a doctor for IBS may be partly related to what happened to you when you were a child. How your parents dealt with any of your childhood complaints can affect the way you deal with them as an adult, according to some studies. Furthermore, the way you deal with your children's complaints can possibly also influence their future behavior in this regard. One study suggested that people with IBS who as children had remained home from school or had received gifts when they were ill were more likely to seek some type of medical care.[2] Our childhoods may continue to mold our behavior throughout our lives. Remember this when dealing with your own children.

HOW IS IBS DIAGNOSED?

Symptoms and Tests

"I have had every test known to mankind, and some of them twice."

"I feel cheated in my diagnosis. IBS is something that I have read that 20% of the population is now being diagnosed with, and I feel as though it is a 'default' diagnosis when no other condition is evident. I do believe that it is possible that I do

indeed have a severe form of IBS, but I also believe that the human body is full of complex processes and that another explanation could have been missed. I feel that a condition as severe and pervasive as mine could not simply be IBS."

We now know that more often than not, people with the typical symptoms of IBS will be found, after tests, to have IBS and not some other sinister condition. It seems likely IBS is a complex disease process that we still poorly understand, but this does not mean we cannot diagnose it easily in many cases. Indeed, your doctor can make a positive diagnosis without tests in most cases![3] There are also "red-flag" complaints that need to be considered here. If you have a red-flag complaint, you should be tested for other conditions. On the other hand, if you have no red-flag features and your symptoms are typical, the chance that tests will find anything is very low (but not zero).

So what are these red-flag complaints? Red-flag complaints are those that strongly suggest that there may be an underlying structural or metabolic problem. Table 2-1 shows a list of red-flag symptoms. If you have lost weight and have

Table 2-1: Red-Flag Symptoms That Suggest You Should See a Doctor
Weight loss (7 pounds or more) without dieting
Increasing difficulty in swallowing
Evidence of bleeding (eg, blood in the stool)
Fatty stool (pale, very smelly, difficult to flush away)
Repeated vomiting
Fever
First onset in older age
Symptoms that awaken you from sleep
Severe diarrhea
Strong family history of cancer

not been dieting, this is a red-flag symptom. Weight loss can have lots of explanations. However, if you have lost significant amounts of weight and have not been trying to diet, you should see a doctor right away. Any bowel bleeding is also a worry. Blood in the stool may just be due to hemorrhoids or some other minor condition. Hemorrhoidal bleeding typically shows as small amounts of bright red blood noticed on wiping or seen on the stool. However, hemorrhoidal bleeding cannot be just assumed unless a doctor has done appropriate testing to exclude serious causes such as a bowel cancer, which while uncommon, can present with bleeding.

Symptoms that occur for the first time when one is over the age of 40 years are generally considered to be an alarm indicator because of the high rate of colon cancer in the United States. Colon cancer rarely presents in people younger than 40 years but unfortunately is not that uncommon in those over 50 years of age. About 5% of Americans who have no family history of colon cancer will develop it in their lifetime; 90% of cases occur in people who are over 50 years of age. It is for this reason that screening of the US population aged 50 years and over for colon cancer is currently recommended whether or not there are any symptoms. Colon cancer can present with absolutely no symptoms initially, but bowel symptoms and abdominal pain or discomfort can be the first warning features. Other features of concern are a clear-cut change in bowel habits, for example, from a normal pattern to diarrhea or constipation, or a sudden unexpected switch from diarrhea to constipation or vice versa.

Many professional societies now recommend a screening evaluation for colon cancer in people aged 50 years and over, even if they have no symptoms. Should you have symptoms and be in this age bracket, you and your doctor should discuss the role of a test to exclude the possibility of any type of colon cancer or a polyp that can grow into colon cancer. If you have a family history of colon cancer, are known to have a colon polyp, or have had long-standing ulcerative colitis or Crohn's disease, then the risk of colon cancer is higher, and you should discuss screening with your doctor. Screening can be done by radiography (x-rays) or preferably by colonoscopy (inserting a type of camera called a colonoscope into the bowel). Colonoscopy (Figure 2-1) is a safe test but, like all invasive medical tests, has the potential for complications even in the very best hands. There can be complications from the medications used to make the test comfortable, such as suppression of breathing or effects on heart function because of a low oxygen rate in the blood; this is why oxygen saturation in the blood is monitored during the procedure. A tear (perforation) in the bowel occurs in up to 2 of 1,000 cases. This complication requires an operation or hospitalization and is therefore potentially very serious. Bleeding from biopsies can also occur but is relatively rare. Cleaning out the colon with laxatives is a routine part of the procedure so that the lining can be seen properly. Furthermore, it is important to

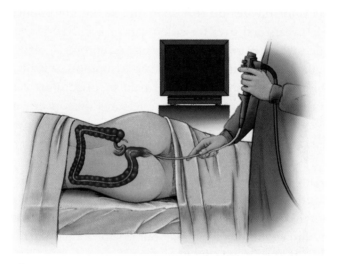

Figure 2-1: Colonoscopy.

clean out the bowel because bacteria in the colon produce concentrations of combustible gases. These gases can explode when a polyp is removed by using diathermy (this is a very rare event now that is not pleasant to think about). You'll be pleased to know that with current bowel preparations, explosions virtually never occur. There can be other very rare complications with endoscopy, even death. It is for this reason that while tests such as endoscopy may be needed, it is very important for you and your doctor to weigh the potential risks and benefits. In striving to help, medicine (whether by tests or treatments) can be harmful.

There are now many jokes about colonoscopy, one of the fastest-rising procedures being done in the United States. The procedure is usually done with the patient under sedation (it can be done without sedation in those with a high pain tolerance), and patients sometimes talk although most just doze. One man reportedly said, "Could you write a note for my wife, saying that my head is in fact not up there?" I can't vouch for the accuracy of the report (and it's my experience that comments such as this do not occur much), but I include it for your interest.

If you have no alarm features, then the pattern of your symptoms will be very helpful in determining whether or not you have clear-cut IBS. A questionnaire is included in this book (Appendix 2) to help you, but you still need to see a doctor to confirm the information. To be diagnosed with having IBS, you must have abdominal discomfort or pain that is associated with an abnormality of the bowels. Typically, the abdominal pain or discomfort is relieved when you open your bowels, at least for a short time. However, not everybody with IBS gets relief when they open their bowels. If your stools change when the pain begins or during periods of pain, becoming looser or harder, this is a strong indicator of IBS. On the other hand, if your stool frequency changes with the pain, either increasing or decreasing, this is also a strong indicator of IBS. The current diagnostic criteria for IBS demand that you have two of these three symptoms, as listed in Table 2-2.

However, as has been said, not everybody with IBS will fulfill these strict diagnostic criteria. If you have abdominal pain and an abnormal bowel habit, you are still likely to have a type of IBS. This likelihood is increased if you also have felt bloated or have noticed that your stomach visually swells, have seen a white slimy material (called mucus) in the stool, or have felt that you cannot completely empty your bowels when you go.

The British are famous for being obsessed with their bowel function, so trust a team in Britain to come up with a scale for grading stools! There are seven grades, based on the appearance of the stool in the toilet bowl (Figure 2-2). This is called

Table 2-2: International (Rome) Diagnostic Criteria* for IBS†

A three-month history of abdominal discomfort or pain that has two of the following three features:

1. Relieved with passing stool
2. Onset associated with a change in frequency of stool
3. Onset associated with a change in form (appearance) of stool

Symptoms that cumulatively support the diagnosis of irritable bowel syndrome:

- Abnormal stool frequency (more than three bowel movements per day or less than three bowel movements per week)
- Abnormal stool form (lumpy/hard or loose/watery stool)
- Abnormal stool passage (straining, urgency, or feeling of incomplete emptying)
- Passage of mucus (white slimy substance)
- Bloating

*In the absence of structural or metabolic abnormalities to explain the symptoms.
†See Appendix 1 for the patient questionnaire.
Adapted from Drossman DA, editor. The functional gastrointestinal disorders. Rome II. 2nd ed. 2000. Available at: http://www.romecriteria.org.

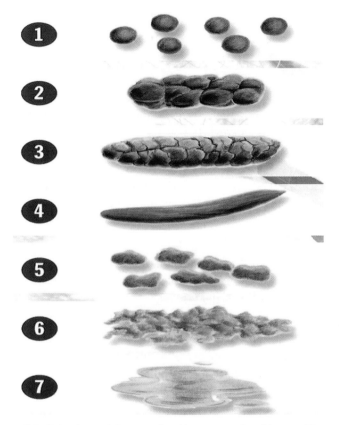

Figure 2-2: Bristol stool form scale. 1) separate hard lumps like nuts (difficult to pass), 2) sausage shaped but lumpy, 3) like a sausage but with cracks on its surface, 4) like a sausage or snake, smooth and soft, 5) soft blobs with clear-cut edges (passed easily), 6) fluffy pieces with ragged edges, a mushy stool, 7) liquid stool.

the Bristol stool form scale, and it is remarkable because it can be used by anyone and measures real changes in the stool. Further, the stool types correlate with "gut transit," indicating if it is long (a "slow gut") or short (a "fast gut").[4] Another team, this time from the United States, developed an instrument that measures the hardness of the stool by applying a pressure device to a stool sample. This turned out to be rather unhelpful; even if the stool feels hard, it is not usually physically harder. Moreover, this is not a particularly fun test to do, and the research (to my knowledge) has not been repeated.[5]

Remember, lots of things can lead to short-term changes in your bowels. If you are pregnant or if it is just before your period, you may notice that you become constipated or have diarrhea, and this is normal. If you have had a hysterectomy, you may sometimes have short-lived bowel symptoms although some women also develop IBS after a hysterectomy. Many people without IBS can have diarrhea for a short time after eating something that upsets their stomach. People with IBS typically feel that their symptoms are worse after they eat certain foods, but this is usually highly variable. If you are traveling, you may develop diarrhea or even constipation (particularly if you are afraid to use some of the terrible public toilets that exist in the world). Of course, traveler's diarrhea can be a short-term problem, but some people will develop IBS after food poisoning or a gastroenteritis attack and will have the condition for life (this topic is discussed further in the next chapter). If you have been confined to bed or have lost weight for other reasons, you may become constipated, and this may have nothing to do with IBS. And, of course, if you are particularly nervous (eg, before a job interview or an examination), then diarrhea is frequent although it usually settles once the stress goes away. In people with IBS, however, bowel function problems do not completely settle after a particular stress but tend to occur intermittently anyway, whether or not there is active stress (although stress may make the problem much worse).

We can now objectively measure abdominal swelling in IBS with a machine (the bloatometer, developed by Dr. Peter Whorwell and colleagues in England; Peter is also a pioneer in research into hypnotherapy for IBS).[6] From measurements with this machine, it is clear that swelling occurs more often later in the day and goes away during the night while sleeping.

There are a number of symptoms that are much more common in people with IBS than in people for whom there is some other structural or organic explanation for their problem. "Organic" can mean inflammation (such as in ulcerative colitis or Crohn's disease) or cancer. For example, in a British study, it was found that patients who complained of (1) relief of pain with a bowel movement, (2) more frequent bowel movements when their pain began, (3) looser stools when their pain began, (4) visible abdominal swelling, (5) feelings of not having completely emptied the bowel, and (6) mucus in the stools were more likely to have IBS than some other disorder.[7] Indeed, 94% of those with IBS had two or more of these six symptoms. The six symptoms that this study report identified are now known as the Manning Criteria, named after Adrian Manning, the lead author of the report and a gastroenterologist in Britain. In the medical literature, there is often reference to the Manning Criteria when the diagnosis of IBS is being considered. Typically, the Manning Criteria refer to two or more of the six symptoms in any combination although some investigators believe you must have three or four of these six symptoms for an accurate diagnosis of IBS. These criteria, however, largely ignored constipation.

Rome Criteria: A New International Standard for IBS
The Manning Criteria were superseded by the international criteria, which are also now called the Rome criteria because all of the consensus meetings to develop the criteria were held in Rome, Italy. The author was fortunate to be a founding member of the coordinating committee that helped develop the criteria for IBS and the other functional gastrointestinal disorders.

The first known English-language description of IBS actually appeared in the early 1800s.[8–10] Indigestion, flatulence, and abdominal pain were recognized as symptoms of a condition having no obvious structural explanation then. In 1849, Dr. Cumming stated, "the bowels are at one time constipated and another lax in the same person…how the disease has two such different symptoms I do not propose to explain."[9] But real scientific interest in IBS began to percolate only just 30 years ago.

The Rome criteria followed an international congress that was held in 1984 in Lisbon, where Professor Albert Torsoli, a distinguished gastroenterologist based in Rome, discussed with Professor Grant Thompson, from Ottawa, Canada, the urgent need for international guidelines for the diagnosis and study of IBS. In 1987, a working team made up of Professors Doug Drossman from the United States, Ken Heaton from the United Kingdom, Gerhard Doteval from Sweden, and Wolfgang Kruis from Germany met and debated about what symptoms identified IBS and could be used to make a diagnosis. After a few days, they finally reached a consensus definition (how much of this was helped by many servings of Italian wine and heated debates over dinner is unclear). The early Rome criteria were then presented at an international congress in Rome in 1988 and published in 1989. Following that meeting, Doug Drossman took the initiative and set up a new committee (of which Grant Thompson and I were members) to classify all of the functional gastrointestinal disorders. Since then, the Rome process has snowballed into a major international effort across all continents. The Rome criteria have gone through a number of iterations, with what is known as the Rome III criteria being the latest version. These sets of criteria each culminate a 4-year effort by a large group of distinguished experts in the field who review the evidence and make recommendations after reaching a consensus (which is not always easy).

I was fortunate to become involved in the Rome process at the invitation of Doug Drossman, at Digestive Diseases Week 1989, a major meeting attended by over 11,000 gastroenterologists. I had just given a lecture on nonulcer dyspepsia, a condition that had been little studied at the time. I still remember Doug striding across the room after the lecture to talk to me about this idea of creating a classification for all the unexplained gastrointestinal disorders in order to try and standardize the field and move it forward. I was enthusiastic about the concept. However, I also remember discussing this with other experts in the field who were almost all highly critical and skeptical. I was advised that the concept of subdividing these disorders on the basis of symptoms would be limiting for researchers in the field and might lead to a general loss of interest. How wrong they were! But I was also naive. I thought that this process would be relatively straightforward. I had my own ideas about what symptoms would be useful and felt that it would not be too difficult to develop a good classification of IBS and other related conditions; here I was wrong. Even today, there remains controversy about the classification although most experts endorse it. The field has become standardized, and there have been substantial advances, in part because of the new classification approach. However, it is very clear that there remains an enormous amount to learn. Only by rigorous research will advances be possible, and as in all fields, research progress will occur in fits and starts, with blind alleys and glimpses of the truth. Nevertheless, this whole area remains particularly exciting as advances continue to occur. The most recent concepts will be summarized in this book for you.

Summing Up: Diagnosis

> *"Another great difference is observable in different constitutions in regard to the evacuation by stool. One man never went but once in a month; another had twelve stools every day for 30 years, and afterwards seven in a day for seven years, and in the meantime did not fall away, but rather grew fat." (William Heberden, 1802)*

So IBS can be diagnosed by simply and carefully considering your complaints. If you see your doctor, simple tests will sometimes be ordered to make sure there is no other explanation for the problem (Table 2-3). For example, a blood count may be taken to make sure there is no evidence of anemia (low hemoglobin), which can occur with lower intestinal bleeding that may not be otherwise obvious. Celiac disease is due to an allergy to the proteins in wheat, rye, and barley products; it is treated by means of a special gluten-free diet that the patient must adhere to for life. Celiac disease may be more common in those with IBS-type symptoms (about 1 in 20 may have it),

Table 2-3: Tests for Suspected Functional Gastrointestinal Disorders

Representative Tests	Conditions Being Screened for
Useful but nonessential tests	
Hematology, ESR, and CRP	Anemia, inflammation
Chemistry panel	Liver dysfunction, kidney disturbance
Thyroid function testing	Thyroid dysfunction (under- or over-active thyroid)
Antigliadin, antiendomysial, transglutaminase antibodies	Celiac disease
Other tests	
Stool test for blood	Bleeding
Flexible sigmoidoscopy	Colitis, cancer
Stool studies (microscopy, microbiology)	Infection (if diarrhea)
Colonoscopy or barium enema (patients > 50 years of age)	Colitis, cancer
Lactose tolerance test	Lactose intolerance
Colonic transit studies	Slow colon (causing severe constipation)
Pelvic floor studies (anorectal manometry)	Muscle problem around the anus (causing severe constipation)

CRP = C-reactive protein; ESR = erythrocyte sedimentation rate.

so your doctor may check blood test results for this possibility.[3] Celiac disease typically causes diarrhea but can sometimes also cause constipation. Your doctor may also consider measuring your thyroid function because people who have an under- or overactive thyroid can present with constipation or diarrhea. An examination of the colon can be done with an endoscope (a special camera) or by radiography. A short endoscope can be used to look at part of the colon (flexible sigmoidoscopy) whereas the whole colon can be examined with a colonoscope. A number of radiographic techniques can now be used to examine the bowel. The traditional approach uses an enema with barium, a thick white paste that can be seen on x-ray films; it allows the lining of the bowel to be seen properly (Figure 2-3). More advanced approaches such as virtual colonoscopy can image the colon and reconstruct it almost as realistically as if a scope had been passed through it (Figure 2-4). However, as has been said above, if there are no other alarm features and the symptoms are absolutely typical of IBS,

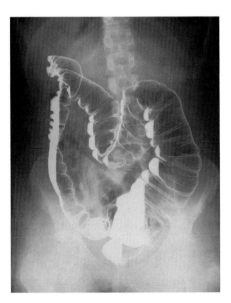

Figure 2-3: Barium enema. There is spasm (narrowing) of part of the colon in this patient with IBS, which disappeared during the test.

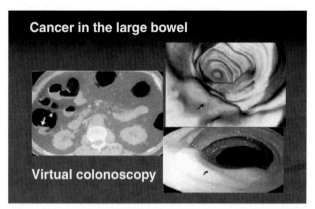

Figure 2-4: Example of images obtained by virtual colonoscopy. Reproduced with permission from Fenlon HM, Nunes DP, Schroy PC III, et al. A comparison of virtual and conventional colonoscopy for the detection of colorectal polyps. N Engl J Med 1999;341:1496–503.

the chance that any of these tests will show a significant abnormality is very small (but not zero).

SO YOU THINK YOU MIGHT HAVE IBS NOW?

"As far as working with your doctor, that's a laugh. My doctor sent me to three different gastroenterologists. Not one of them examined me in any way and were not interested in return visits. Wrote out some prescription for tablets I'd told them I had already tried. Easy money earned and are not interested in how you feel. No bedside manners at all."

If your symptoms are worrying you, it would be wise to see a doctor to make sure IBS is the diagnosis. This will also give you some peace of mind about the condition. Self-diagnosis is sometimes difficult and is certainly not recommended. Unfortunately, some people don't get a satisfactory answer, but finding a good physician to work with you can help. Get a second opinion if you are still worried or dissatisfied. Institutions

Date	Time	Abdominal pain or discomfort (and how long)?	Stool passed (hard, soft, normal)	Bloating	Related to any food?	Any Stress?	Any medications taken?

Diet:
List items and times

Breakfast

Lunch

Dinner

Snacks

Exercise
List: walk, run, bike, other – and times

Figure 2-5: Example of a daily symptom diary for patients with irritable bowel syndrome.

like the Mayo Clinic have clinics staffed by specialists for diagnosing and treating IBS, so consider this option as well.

Your doctor will want to know when your symptoms began, exactly what they are, whether they have changed recently, and what are you taking for them now or have taken in the past. Consider keeping a diary in which you write down all the symptoms each day for 2 weeks, including when they occurred and their relationship to meals or bowel movements (Figure 2-5). On the other hand, bringing a box load of material downloaded from the Internet won't usually impress your doctor, but having a summary of any past tests, if available, is very useful.

Once you have been given a diagnosis of IBS, what can be done? To understand the options, you also need to know why IBS might occur and how you can take control of this problem and treat it effectively. This is what the rest of this book is about. Make the journey with me as we explore the mysterious workings of the bowel and what can be done to help make it work better for you.

Take-Home Messages

- IBS is a common and real problem; you are not alone!
- IBS can be accurately diagnosed by your doctor without tests in most cases.
- For IBS, tests are used to rule out a surprise cause for the symptoms.
- Even if you have an abnormal test result, you can still have IBS plus another problem; your doctor can sort this out for you.
- Gastroenterologists (specialists in stomach and bowel problems) have expertise in doing tests and interpreting symptoms if there is any uncertainty.

CHAPTER 3

WHY DOES IRRITABLE BOWEL SYNDROME OCCUR?

"Discovery consists of looking at the same thing as everyone else does and thinking something different." (Albert Szent-Györgyi, 1937 Nobel Prize winner in physiology and medicine)

How do the stomach and small and large bowels work? Essentially, the stomach and bowels exist so that we can turn food into a usable fuel for all of the cells in our body. To do this, we need to be able to adequately absorb fluids as well as digest our food. This in turn requires the bowel to propel material it takes in throughout the digestive tube.

NORMAL ANATOMY AND FUNCTION

It is a joy to eat! As Woody Allen and Marshall Brickman have said, "My brain, it's my second favorite organ." Some may argue about what their first choice might be, but it seems to me that if you cannot eat, life is just miserable, so I vote for my stomach and bowels.

The anatomy of the gut (stomach, small bowel, and large bowel) is shown in Figure 3-1. The esophagus is a swallowing tube; the lower two-thirds of the esophagus are made up of muscle that reflexly propels liquids and solids into the stomach even if we are standing on our heads. This movement is referred to as a peristaltic reflex because it is not under conscious control after the food enters the top part of the esophagus. There is a muscle at the lower end of the esophagus (called the lower esophageal sphincter) that normally relaxes as the fluid or food moves down the esophagus. Although the mouth is above the rest of the esophagus when we stand up, gravity is not at all important in moving material through this tube.

The stomach is situated in the upper left-hand side of the abdominal cavity. The stomach itself is more than just a food

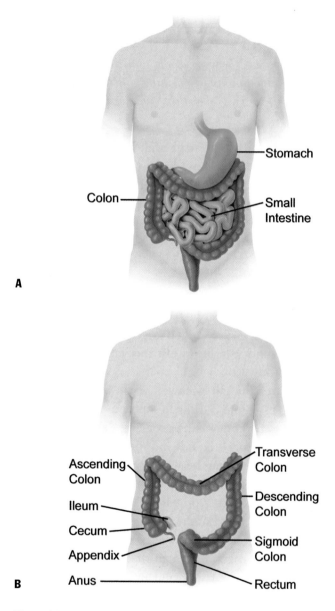

A

B

Figure 3-1: Anatomy of the stomach, small intestine, and colon inside the abdomen.

reservoir. When you eat a meal, the top part of the stomach (called the fundus) relaxes to prevent the pressure in the stomach from rising excessively. This relaxation of the stomach allows you to feel satisfied yet not uncomfortable after you eat. If this reflex response becomes abnormal, then you may become very uncomfortable after eating and may be unable to finish a normal-sized meal; this symptom is generally called early satiety (or satiation) in the medical literature.

The stomach grinds the food eaten into smaller particles and squirts out hydrochloric acid, which helps to sterilize the contents. The acid would burn your skin, but it doesn't normally burn the stomach lining. The stomach empties relatively slowly, in a carefully orchestrated process. This allows the food to enter the small bowel in controlled amounts so that it can be handled more easily. If food passes rapidly from the stomach into the small bowel, the bowel becomes suddenly distended, and this can cause weakness and sweating after eating (referred to as dumping syndrome). So while the stomach may fill rapidly, it adapts so that stomach swelling does not cause symptoms, the small bowel is not overfilled, and digestion is allowed to occur normally in the small bowel (the stomach does not essentially digest the food).

Normal emptying of a meal from the stomach takes up to 4 hours, with the bulk of the meal leaving by 2 hours. Women empty their stomachs more slowly than men as a group. Stomach emptying also depends partly on the type of food eaten. Liquids like water empty fast while liquids containing sugar empty more slowly. Fatty foods are slowest in leaving the stomach; protein-enriched foods leave somewhat more quickly whereas sugar (carbohydrate-rich) foods leave the stomach most quickly. This is why some people drink milk or cream before cocktails, as the fat slows the stomach emptying of alcohol so more can be taken without feeling drunk. Through nerve cells, the top part of the small bowel, called the duodenum, is able to sense the contents coming from the stomach (a bit like tasting them). These receptors in the duodenum then (through reflex nerve pathways) slow stomach emptying. The brain can also directly affect stomach emptying. For example, fear can slow stomach emptying whereas being excited can increase the speed of emptying. For this reason, a high-fat diet or being fearful can make some symptoms arising from the stomach worse because of aggravation of an already slow rate of stomach emptying.

The small bowel (or small intestine) is about 30 feet long and goes from the end of the stomach to the beginning of the large intestine described below. It lies in the center of the abdominal cavity and is divided into three parts (duodenum, jejunum, and ileum). Here food is mixed, digested, and absorbed, and waste material is passed on to the colon. The large intestine, or colon, is 6 feet long and normally curls around the small bowel and then passes down and around the outer area of the abdominal cavity, ending up at the anus. The colon is a storage organ; it allows excessive fluid to be absorbed from the waste (stool). The colon retains stool (it is hoped) until it is socially acceptable to expel it (see page 86).

The basic unit of intestinal propulsion is the peristaltic reflex (see Figure 8-1 on page 154). Any distention of the bowel (eg, by food) stimulates a reflex response that leads to a contraction that pushes the food down, followed by relaxation of the bowel below the food so that it can move forward without difficulty. This is all an unconscious process. Within the stomach and small bowel, there is an electrical rhythm because of the presence of special electrical signaling cells called interstitial cells of Cajal (ICC). In the presence of the electrical rhythm, the muscle can contract. However, this is a flexible situation because the nerves in the bowel wall are able to inhibit the muscle cells that are being activated. This allows the bowel to unconsciously fine-tune the movement of material through it. You can think of the bowel as a fine tuned sports car; the engine is on all of the time (the electrical rhythm), but unless the clutch (the muscle cell) is engaged, nothing moves forward. The electrical signalling cells can be lost or damaged leading to chronic constipation.

The bowel is under control both locally, from what is called the enteric nervous system, and centrally, from the brain. The enteric nervous system is a series of nerve cell families that sends fibers to muscle in the bowel as well as to the lining of the bowel. The enteric nervous system also can sense signals from the lining, as some sensory nerves connect up the system. These nerve networks contain hard-wired programs ("gut software") that coordinate set patterns of motor activity when you are fasting and after you eat a meal. For example, one of these programs is called the migrating motor complex (MMC). The MMC is a pattern of regular muscle contractions that move down the bowel, cleaning out its contents. This is why the MMC is also called the "intestinal housekeeper." Giant waves can occur ("power propulsion") that can cause pain (cramps) and diarrhea.

The brain interacts with the bowel through the autonomic nervous system, which comprises the vagus and pelvic nerves (referred to as the parasympathetic nervous system) and nerves from the spinal cord (called the sympathetic nervous system). The vagus and pelvic nerves send information to the brain concerning the movement of muscle and bowel content. On the other hand, the nerves in the sympathetic nervous system send information to the brain about swelling of the bowel or inflammation in the bowel that may cause pain. The brain sends signals to the bowel through the autonomic nervous system too, so it's a two-way street. The brain can also finely regulate the bowel in other ways. For example, a hormone called corticotropin-releasing factor (CRF) can alter bowel activity and is released during stress from the brain. Drugs that alter CRF are being developed for treating IBS. As you can see, if you are stressed or upset, your bowel often reacts through this complex system. No wonder one often experiences diarrhea before an ordeal or a big test (like your wedding day or an important school exam)!

A number of bowel hormones also are important in normal control of digestion. Gastrin is released from the stomach when food enters it, which in turn stimulates special cells (called parietal cells) in the upper part of the stomach (the fundus) to secrete gastric acid. Cholecystokinin (CCK), another hormone released from the small bowel, leads to contraction of the gall bladder (the organ that concentrates bile for digestion) as well as to the secretion of enzymes from the pancreas (also for digestion). Motilin is a small-bowel hormone that "turns on" the MMC. There is some evidence that CCK may be abnormally released in IBS although this is not certain. Whether other bowel hormones are important in IBS remains unclear.

CAUSE OF IBS

> "I have had a 'sensitive stomach' since I can remember. My mother is the same. I guess I never thought too much about it until my university years, when my social life, as well as my studies, began to suffer. I finally decided to go to the doctor, concerned there was something seriously wrong with me. Nearly 2 years and five doctors later, I had a diagnosis—irritable bowel syndrome—but they still couldn't tell me what to do about it."

There are a number of different theories about the underlying cause of IBS. Now that we have reviewed some of the relevant anatomy and physiology, it is time to turn to what may be abnormal in those who suffer with IBS. The first thing to make clear is there is no change in anatomy in IBS. The bowel of a person with IBS looks completely normal on an x-ray film or through an endoscope. Don't be upset or surprised by this fact. This doesn't mean it is normal, but one needs better tools to find the abnormalities; so the bowel's looking normal in IBS does not mean that it is functioning normally in IBS. As you can appreciate now, the bowel is a very complex organ that has a number of different control mechanisms in place. Subtle abnormalities of the nerves or muscles can lead to decreased or increased bowel function that in turn can lead to the symptoms exprienced by people with IBS. The reason why it is important to fully understand the abnormalities is that this is the only way of devising effective new approaches to fix the underlying problems. Unfortunately, a clear picture of the full range of abnormalities in IBS is not yet available. There are lots of hints, and there is no doubt in my mind that IBS is a real disease, but much more needs to be learned.

The current views of potential mechanisms and some evidence for the abnormalities are presented in the following section.

Do We Know the Cause of IBS?

What is the cause of IBS? Unfortunately, no one yet knows. However, knowledge is increasing, and it seems likely that with more research, it will be possible to identify the true cause in the near future. Indeed, it is likely that this is not one disease but several diseases; hence, there will be several different causes. The body can react to damaging stimuli in only a small number of ways. For example, when you get traveler's diarrhea because of an infection, the bowel has a limited

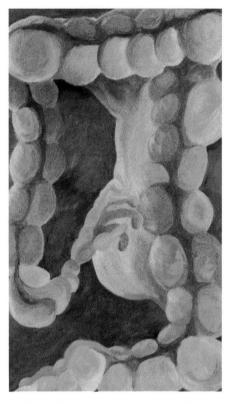

Attack of the Irritable Bowel, from the International Foundation for Functional Gastronintestinal Disorders (IFFGD) Art of IBS Collection. Printed with permission from the IFFGD (© 2004 IFFGD).

response to this in terms of the symptoms experienced. However, a number of different bacterial and viral organisms can cause very similar bowel symptoms. The same may well be true for IBS; hence, we need to look for a number of different causes. The hints from research today suggest that there will indeed be quite a few to find.

It seems to me that IBS is a real disease. We are learning that we can find abnormalities if we look hard enough, so be reassured that IBS is not some imagined condition or mysterious entity that will never be unraveled.

Can I Inherit IBS?

Until recently, the idea that IBS might have a genetic component was not considered at all. However, important work done by some of my colleagues and myself, as well as by other expert groups from around the world, suggest that IBS likely has a real genetic component. Some of the first hints that this was the case came from work from the Mayo Clinic, where it was observed that IBS tended to run in families.[1] Of course, diseases can run in families because of similar environments, such as diet, as well as for genetic reasons. Hence, this work did not answer the question of whether genes were definitely important although it gave a hint. The next pieces of evidence came from studies of twins.[2,3] Twins are excellent models for studying disease because identical twins share exactly the same genes whereas nonidentical twins share 50% of the same genes (just like brothers and sisters do). Hence, if you are able to show that a certain disease is more likely to occur in an identical twin as compared with a nonidentical twin, this suggests that genes are contributing to that process if the environment has otherwise been similar. Using this classic type of approach to study genetic disease, my colleagues and I undertook the first study of twins to evaluate IBS, in Sydney, Australia.[2] We showed that genes indeed appeared to explain just over 50% of the development of IBS. This was exciting, and further work from the United States has supported these findings although the genetic component may be less than was initially suggested by the Sydney study.[3]

Attempts to find possible genes that might contribute to IBS are now ongoing. New results here have been very exciting. For example, Dr. Gerald Holtmann led an important effort, in collaboration with myself, that identified one particular gene (*GNB3* polymorphism) that was linked to nonulcer dyspepsia and possibly IBS.[4] This was important because the gene being studied regulates a large series of different bodily processes, which may account for the fact that IBS doesn't just affect the bowel but can affect other organ systems. Much more work is needed to confirm these initial observations. Other genes may also be important in IBS, and great efforts are going into research in this field. Some of these genes regulate the inflammatory process[5] whereas others regulate serotonin reuptake (an important chemical regulator of nerve transmission, including peristalsis) or other key nervous system functions.[6,7] This is most exciting because if all the major genes that contribute to IBS can be identified, it seems likely that new tests and new treatments may become available soon.

Can Infection Cause IBS?

In a classic study from the United Kingdom in the 1960s, about 1 in 5 people with IBS reported having developed their symptoms after some kind of infection, such as stomach flu or traveler's diarrhea.[8] Most people obviously recover from these acute illnesses without any problems, but this early work suggested that some people, for whatever reason, continue to have bowel symptoms and that these symptoms could persist over the long term.

Studies in the last few years have further evaluated this issue, and it is clear that this has led to important new insights. First of all, after an acute bowel infection from bacteria (such as *Campylobacter* or *Salmonella*), a small minority (perhaps 10%) of patients do not recover but continue to have chronic bowel symptoms with all the features of IBS.[9,10] There are certain people who are more likely to develop this postinfection IBS than are other people. For example, people who are naturally more anxious seem to be at higher risk although the reason for this is unclear. It is possible that the genes that may predispose someone to be more anxious than another person could also predispose that person to be more likely to have IBS. There may be other explanations too, but this link between the bowel and the brain is quite striking and potentially very important.

It is also clear that abnormalities are seen when biopsy specimens from the bowels of some people who develop this postinfection IBS are examined under a microscope. Biopsy specimens from the rectum (the bottom end of the large bowel) of patients with postinfectious IBS have shown an increased presence of inflammatory cells (which invade the lining to mop up infections and then persist). A splinter in your toe that you fail to remove promptly attracts lots of inflammatory cells that cause redness, pain, and swelling; even if you remove the splinter, the inflammation may persist for a while before clearing and the tenderness may linger. Inflammation present in the bowel can also lead to abnormal stimulation of nerve cells that might cause pain; even if the inflamation eventually goes away, the nerve cells may remain abnormally excitable, resulting in the pain persisting.[10] This information is largely based on experiments in animals but probably applies to us too.

The inflammatory changes in IBS are very subtle. They were noticed only when the cells were actually counted; indeed, the pathologists who looked at these samples routinely called them normal at first. However, when the cells are counted, there are obviously an increased number in some of those with symptoms of IBS as compared to those who do not have this problem. Hence, some people with IBS actually have a true but subtle inflammatory bowel disease (Figure 3-2). This also has important implications because some people may respond to specific antiinflammatory agents that block certain actions of the cells. However, antiinflammatory agents have not yet been shown to work in IBS patients and are not routinely recommended at this time.

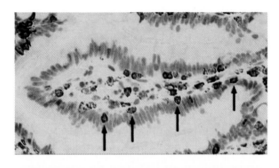

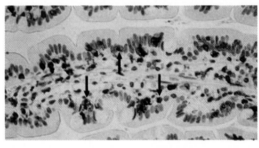

Figure 3-2: In the upper small intestine, full-thickness biopsy specimens in 9 out of 10 patients with IBS showed low-grade infiltration of lymphocytes in the nerve (myenteric) plexus. This was increased over control tissue. An example of one control subject (top figure) and one IBS patient (bottom figure) is shown. With permission from Tornblom et al. *Gastroenterology.* 2002 Dec;123(6):1972-9.

Processing Signals in the Brain:
Are Some People's Wires Crossed?

You catch your hand in the car door; it hurts! But your brain has to process the signal from the hand for you to feel the pain. If the sensory nerves carrying these signals from the hand to the brain were damaged, you would not feel pain. Similarly, you would not feel any sensations in your stomach or abdomen if the brain did not process the signals it was receiving. When the pathways that send the signals out from the bowel to the brain are cut in animal experiments, the animals do not feel pain, for example, from the bowel area being stretched. Similarly, the brain is able to actually signal the bowel and turn down the information being sent up to it for processing. Hence, the brain is able to partly control any type of pain or discomfort although this is an unconscious process.

There has been a lot of interest in looking at the brains of people with IBS to see whether their processing of signals from the bowel could be different from such processing in those who don't have IBS. Indeed, the studies now suggest that the processing of such signals is different in IBS.[11-13] From data obtained with sophisticated scanning techniques such as positron emission tomography (PET) and magnetic resonance imaging (MRI), it is clear that the blood flow to certain key brain areas that process pain signals "lights up" more in people with IBS as compared to healthy people (see Figure 3-3).

You can see that the brain is a key organ in the experience of IBS, as it is in the experience of any chronic painful illness. The experience of IBS will therefore be affected by other factors that influence brain activity. Some of these factors must include early life experiences as well as any problems with stress, which is so common in the population. If you are predisposed to increase the processing of unpleasant stimuli, this may in turn lead to repeated negative thoughts or to increased anxiety and depression, and thereby worsen bowel symptoms in a vicious circle that aggravates IBS. This probably applies only to some people with IBS and not to others, but it is important to recognize this if it is present because the type of treatment can be tailored accordingly. Abnormal processing of signals reaching the brain may be why certain drugs such as antidepressants can work in people with IBS. It may also be why (based on the best available evidence) psychological treatment such as hypnotherapy is useful for people with IBS.

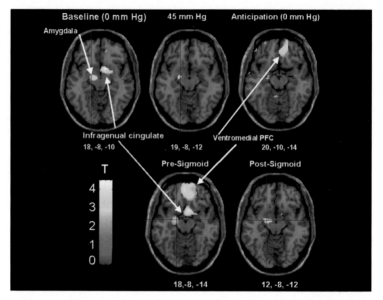

Figure 3-3: The part of the brain called the amygdala in IBS is important in pain processing. The drug alosetron decreases blood flow in this area in response to stretching the colon with a balloon. This may mean the drug reduces pain by signaling the brain. Reprinted from Chang L. Brain responses to visceral and somatic stimuli in irritable bowel syndrome: a central nervous system disorder? *Gastroenterology Clinics of North America* 2005;34:271-9 with permission from Elsevier.

Sexual and Physical Abuse

This is a difficult and sensitive area, but research suggests that a history of having been abused as a child or as an adult can predispose you to IBS.[14,15] In a study we did in a US community, 40% of women and 10% of men reported a history of some type of abuse, a frighteningly high rate.[15] Certainly, only some people with IBS have a history of any type of abuse, but such a history is about twice as common in people who have developed IBS than in people who don't have the condition.

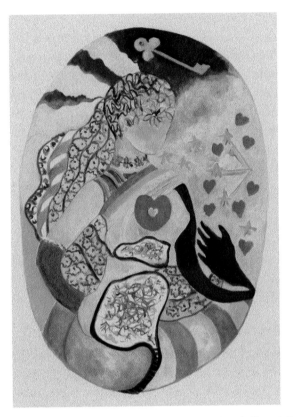

The IBS Anxiety Experience, from the International Foundation for Functional Gastrointestinal Disorders (IFFGD) Art of IBS Collection. Printed with permission from the IFFGD (© 2004 IFFGD).

What is abuse? There is no straightforward answer, and the word is open to various interpretations. Certain types of abuse are very obvious whereas other types of abuse are more subtle. At the extreme end of the spectrum is rape, attempted rape, and severe physical abuse with beatings. People with IBS do not commonly report this although, again, such events are sadly still more common in IBS patients. Other events are classified as abusive by some people but not by others.

Bullying at school, for example, is a form of abuse, but some people are not affected by it in any serious way whereas others are. Similarly, being touched inappropriately in the work environment might be considered a form of sexual abuse by some whereas others will not be particularly concerned (even if they should be).

If you have been abused or feel that you may have been abused, this is worth discussing with your physician. Sometimes revealing the experience and talking it over can be very helpful in terms of learning to manage your IBS. Not everyone who has been abused wants to talk about it, and that is reasonable, but you should consider seeking the counsel of your physician here. A small minority of people who have undergone any abuse will benefit from formal counseling, particularly if the events are still intruding into their lives in a major way.

ABNORMAL BOWEL SENSATION

As discussed elsewhere in this book, the nervous system of the bowel (the enteric nervous system) controls the functions of the bowel locally; this is not under conscious control. There are lots of different reflex pathways that control the contraction of the bowel muscle, the secretion of fluid into the bowel, the blood flow to the bowel, and the feeling arising from the bowel. The enteric nervous system connects with other nerve pathways, so this is a very complex network. The nerve cells themselves contain different chemicals, or even gases (neurotransmitters) that allow the nerves to essentially "talk" to each other. These transmitters include substances such as 5-hydroxytryptamine (serotonin), acetylcholine, opioids, somatostatin, substance P, nitric oxide, and vasoactive intestinal polypeptide. I know these names are mouthfuls, but they just reflect the complexity of the system. What's more, nerves often contain more than one neurotransmitter. This is why a number of the newer drugs target neurotransmitter function in order to potentially benefit the patient with IBS. There are many serotonin receptors that, when in contact with serotonin, lead to different effects, and serotonin appears to be particularly important in IBS, based on what we know today. For example, drugs that stimulate the serotonin (type 4) receptor (such as tegaserod [Zelnorm]) tend to make material move faster through the bowel and also may reduce the transmission of sensation from the bowel to the brain. Similarly, drugs that block the serotonin (type 3) receptor (such as alosetron [Lotronex]) also reduce signals going from the bowel to the brain but tend to slow down the movement of material through the bowel. These drugs therefore work on different symptoms of IBS and can also have different side effects in IBS patients (see Chapter 8).

There is overwhelming evidence that in IBS, the bowel is more sensitive than normal.[16,17] How do we know this? Well, if you take a biopsy specimen from the lining of the bowel through an endoscope, the patient will feel absolutely nothing when the biopsy sample is taken because there are no sensory nerves in the lining of the bowel that can feel pain (unlike the skin, where one will feel pain). If a balloon is placed in the bowel and blown up, the person will feel this if the balloon is blown up large enough, even if he or she is normal, because this will stretch the muscle layers where the nerve receptors for pain exist. However, if you have IBS and a balloon is placed in your bowel, you are more likely to feel the balloon when it is less distended compared with healthy people. This increased bowel sensitivity means the brain is more likely to be flooded with signals from the bowel, which is probably important in developing the disease. Drugs that block bowel sensitivity have now been developed, and some have reached the clinic (as will be discussed later).

ABNORMAL BOWEL CONTRACTIONS

In the past, spasm of the bowel was considered to be an important abnormality in IBS because it was thought that this could explain the pain of the condition. This theory (called a hypothesis in science) led to a large number of studies investigating whether the motor functions of the bowel, which move material through it, are abnormal in IBS.[18,19] However, the results have been inconsistent, probably because motor function in the bowel, while not normal in IBS, is not the major cause of the symptoms. It is true that people with diarrhea and IBS tend to have a faster movement of material, particularly through the small bowel and colon. Similarly, people with constipation and IBS, as a group, tend to have a slower movement of material through the small bowel and colon. In IBS, however, the speed of movement tends to vary from day to day and from week to week, and so these abnormalities are not particularly consistent.

ABNORMAL HORMONE RELEASE

The bowel releases a number of different hormones that control some of its functions. For example, when you eat a fatty meal, the hormone cholecystokinin (CCK) is released from the small bowel. CCK contracts the gallbladder and also stimulates the secretion of enzymes from the pancreas, which aids absorption. CCK also has a number of other complex effects, including making you feel full after a meal and possibly altering the movement of material through the small bowel and colon.[19] This has led to some interest in drugs that may block the receptors that are activated by hormones such as CCK, and such drugs may have a role in IBS treatment in the future. However, the hormonal control of the bowel is very complex, and the exact importance of hormones in terms of IBS is unknown. While IBS is more common in women than in men, for example, it doesn't appear that the effect of female sex hormones on bowel function explains this difference (although this is a fruitful area for future investigation).[20]

SUMMING UP

It is clear that IBS is a real condition with real abnormalities that can be demonstrated by careful studies. A number of investigators have pioneered examination of the bowel and the brain in IBS and are studying potential predisposing conditions, such as genes and the early environment. Much more needs to be learned because if we can fully understand the causes of IBS, we will be able to more sensibly intervene in the condition. Still, the findings in the last few years are very exciting and suggest that we will be able to do much more for IBS sufferers in the near future.

Take-Home Messages

- The bowel is complex, but much is known about its normal function.
- IBS is a real disease but may arise from a variety of causes.
- IBS runs in some families; this may be due to genes, environment, or both.
- Stress can aggravate IBS but may not be the main cause.
- We will unlock the causes of IBS; it is only a matter of time—and funding! This will lead to better treatments and possibly a cure.

TAKING CONTROL: WHAT TREATMENTS REALLY WORK?

"Be careful about reading health books. You may die of a misprint." (Mark Twain, 1835–1910)

"An expert is a person who has made all the mistakes that can be made in a very narrow field." (Niels Bohr, 1885–1962)

There is a barrage of information out there on different approaches to treating irritable bowel disease (IBS) and related conditions. Just try an Internet search on the topic; those who have not done so will be amazed at the number of sites that seem to cover the area after just a few clicks. For example, one Web site found with a Google search is entitled "Beating IBS." The author is purportedly a patient who has developed a self-help program that can be purchased for a small sum and that (according to the author) is guaranteed to cure the problem in most people. A number of testimonials support his claims. So the question is, "is this the answer?" Another Web site talks about irritable bowel relief with 100% guaranteed results for an all-natural colon-cleaning product. The trouble is that there are a large number of other sites that make similar claims although most recommend very different sorts of treatment approaches. They, too, have good testimonials. Do all these treatments work? If so, why does it often seem so hard to get better? So how will you know that something could work? How do you know that what you are being told is the truth? Should you believe "the experts" on the net, television, or radio? This is where science can help.

You need to be able to take control here. There is an enormous amount of information out there; some of it is absolute nonsense, and some of it is truly useful. The fact that someone is marketing a product does not mean that what that person says about the product is true (or false).

Furthermore, testimonials alone are not of much value. The fact that one person got better on some kind of treatment for IBS does not mean that the treatment really works. Any benefit of treatment could be due to all sorts of reasons, including the fact that the person's IBS just naturally got better (which can happen in up to one-third of IBS sufferers, without any treatment) or because of what is called the *placebo effect*.

WHAT IS THE PLACEBO EFFECT?

"The art of medicine consists of amusing the patient while nature cures the disease." (Voltaire, 1694-1778)

The word "placebo" means "I shall be pleasing" in Latin. In essence, a placebo is considered to be an inert substance (a sugar pill) that is of apparent therapeutic benefit when taken by a patient. For 200 years, the deliberate prescription of pills that had no action (sugar or dummy pills) was considered a standard part of medicine. However, in more recent years, the use of a placebo has been considered to be deceiving. Indeed, Thomas Jefferson referred to placebos as "a pious fraud." In 1982, Dr. Howard Brody called the placebo, "the lie that heals." Much of what will be summarized here comes from a wonderful review of placebos by Prof. Grant Thompson that appeared in the *American Journal of Gastroenterology*,[1] to which you should go for more details.

The invention of the randomized controlled trial led to real interest in the science behind the placebo effect. The use of a placebo in clinical trials dates from 1938, in a study of cold vaccines in which inert controls were used. Prior to the 1940s, no one seriously thought about always including comparisons of a proposed active treatment with an inert substance. For drugs that have very dramatic results, such as penicillin in the treatment of pneumonia, a placebo-controlled trial is not needed;

either the patient lives or dies, and if almost everybody with certain infections will die without penicillin (as used to be the case), then the benefit of giving the drug to patients is absolutely obvious. However, many drugs, such as cholesterol-lowering agents or blood pressure pills, have much more subtle benefits. Indeed, many treatments have been greeted with enormous enthusiasm by doctors and patients, only to be found, when subjected to a study comparing them with placebo, to be no better than the placebo (and therefore useless). Even worse, some of these treatments caused harm rather than benefit, and so their use was disastrous.

Those who try to sell effective treatments on the Internet and elsewhere thrive on the placebo response! They rely on the fact that this response can be quite high in people with IBS (up to 70% of people actually obtain a short-term benefit from taking almost anything that they might believe in). In this way, many charlatans make a truly great living. Interestingly, the placebo response may last for a long time. Some recent studies comparing new drugs with placebo in IBS over a 1-year period have indicated that the placebo response in those who got better was maintained for an amazing 12-month period. Therefore, placebos can have even long-term benefits for some people. If only we could harvest this response to help you and others with this problem! Hence, research in this area continues.

The How and Why of the Placebo Response

We know from studies already reviewed in this book that the brain plays an important role in IBS. Indeed, dysfunction of certain brain centers may be one of the primary underlying abnormalities in IBS, at least in some people. We also know that the brain can suppress (or "down-regulate") signals coming up from the bowel. If the correct areas in the brain can be activated, the abnormal signals sent to the brain from the bowel can be reduced, and symptoms can thus potentially be made to go away. One way to potentially activate these centers is to truly believe that a treatment really works.

There have been some interesting scientific studies of what predicts a good placebo response although the facts are still somewhat murky. However, the color of a pill can influence the placebo response. For example, blue pills can be depressing whereas pink pills can elevate a person's mood.[2] Larger pills may have more benefit than smaller ones. The experience of being given a pill by a healer is more effective than taking the same pill received by mail. Someone perceived as a healer giving a placebo is more effective at improving a patient than someone perceived as not being a healer. Intelligence does not influence this response at all! The placebo response can vary in an individual; it can be effective at one time and ineffective at another time in the same person. Surgery can induce a placebo response. For example, surgeons will sometimes remove an abdominal organ such as the gallbladder or uterus because they suspect that it is the cause of the symptoms. Even though it becomes very clear later on that the organ was not responsible, the operation itself can still induce a sustained benefit in some people for a period of months at least. Perhaps this accounts for some surgeons' persistent belief in the results of some truly unnecessary surgery. The fact is that unnecessary surgery is often undertaken in IBS cases, and any short-term benefits that occur with such surgery probably reflect this placebo response.

Exactly why the placebo response occurs remains to be fully explained; the brain is still a mysterious organ despite all our probing to date. In conditions under which stress may be important, the placebo response may be greater perhaps because the brain is able to shut down the stress response and reduce the secretion of the important hormone corticotropin-releasing factor (CRF). Drugs that may benefit people with

IBS and other conditions related to stress by blocking the effects of CRF are currently in development. Some of the placebo response is explained by natural fluctuation in IBS. This occurs in many chronic yet intermittent diseases; natural remission will induce what appears to be a placebo response if some kind of pill has been given when the disease is already beginning to get better. Peptic ulcers have seemingly healed on placebo for this reason, as they come and go naturally.

Patients' expectations may also be critical. If you expect to have a certain response, based on your memory of such events and natural conditioning, this may occur. For example, the effects of coffee or alcohol on performance partly depend on what a person expects will occur. In IBS, a local anesthetic given in the rectum can reduce pain from inflating a balloon; verbally suggesting that a particular treatment worked better increased the response to a dummy preparation that contained no anesthetic.[3] A very interesting experiment with 56 medical students supports the importance of this expectation factor.[2] Students in the class were randomly put into four groups; students each were given one blue pill, two blue pills, one pink pill, or two pink pills. All of these students were advised that these pills would have certain effects; the blue pills were said to be sedating, and the pink pills stimulating. About two-thirds of the group were more drowsy with the blue pill. However, all the pills were placebos. Interestingly, two pills had more effect than one. We can all be taken in by the placebo response!

We can also be conditioned to respond to different approaches. Ivan Pavlov, a Russian scientist, was the first to demonstrate in animals that conditioning occurs. Pavlov was astounded when he found that dogs strapped into a harness began to salivate before they were given any meat powder. Prior to this, the dogs had been strapped in and were given meat powder to make them salivate. It seemed they had learned to directly associate being strapped in with salivating. Using the same approach, Pavlov next taught the dogs to salivate to the sound of a bell. He would ring the bell and give meat powder to induce salivation; after a short while, just ringing the bell was enough to make the dogs salivate. Humans can be similarly conditioned. Just like Pavlov's dogs, you can learn to be fearful of something if it is associated with an unpleasant experience. Perhaps as children, some of us have also been conditioned to believe that being given a medicine really is comforting and helpful. Hence, we may essentially learn to be placebo responders. Some may learn better than others, and this may explain why the placebo response works well only in some people and not in others. Such a response could be mediated by a reduction in stress and therefore a change in the brain that subsequently leads to improvement in the IBS symptoms being experienced, even though very abnormal signaling from the bowel continues.

The placebo response may be further influenced by one's cultural background. It is widely believed in different cultures that certain treatments will heal or harm, and this can lead to effects on the human condition. For example, aboriginal people in Australia retain to this day a deep-rooted cultural belief that a hex from a medicine man can be lethal. I remember, as a young doctor in Australia, looking after an aboriginal man in the infectious disease unit who had unexplained high-grade fevers; he had been hexed by "the pointing of the bone." Despite all of the marvels of modern medical technology, no cause was ever found for this man's symptoms; he deeply believed that his illness was a result of the hex put on him, and he died. Whether the hex was the cause or not, the negative impact of a belief clearly affected the management of the problem. (A negative placebo response is called the "nocebo" effect.) Religious belief can also heal. Look at the faith healers who heal on television, with remarkable apparent benefit. This positive force may possibly be linked to the mysterious placebo response in medicine discussed above.

Science is delving deeper into the placebo response all of the time. We know that in the brain, there are a number of nerve pathways that use opiates as nerve pathway transmitters. Indeed, the placebo response to pain can be reversed by using an opiate antagonist medication, suggesting that opiate pathways partly mediate the placebo response, at least for pain.[4] So the placebo response is real, not imagined. Efforts to look at factors that improve or promote this response and may help us to amplify them are under way. As a physician, I know that the doctor-patient interaction can be very positive (or negative) and that part of this positive effect is likely the placebo response. Hence, the placebo response is not unimportant, nor should it be ignored.

Example of the Placebo Response: Unnecessary Surgery

A medical student was once quoted as saying, "The only thing that I learned during my surgery clerkship is that I am never going to have elective surgery." This is an exaggeration, of course, but if you are someone with IBS, think about the statement carefully. One of the disadvantages of going to doctors for management is they will look hard for a possible cause for your symptoms and will sometimes uncover medical problems that in fact have absolutely nothing to do with the pain or bowel dysfunction. A good example is examination of the gallbladder for gallstones. It is very easy to blame the gallbladder for IBS symptoms. Indeed, many people walking around have "silent" gallstones that will never ever cause them any trouble. Gallstones can cause abdominal pain sometimes, however.

Also, abdominal pain can occur when the gallbladder doesn't function properly.

We now know that people with IBS have three times the rate of gallbladder surgery as compared with the rate for people in the normal population in the United States who present for medical care.[5] This means that a very large number of gallbladder operations for IBS are almost certainly unnecessary. The same goes for many appendectomies, hysterectomies, and back operations in people with IBS. The trouble is, once you have had your abdomen opened by a surgeon, adhesions develop, which may cause other problems, and there can occassionally be complications from the surgery itself that can add to the struggle. It is true that sometimes, people with IBS do get better for a while after surgery, which indeed encourages the surgeon and the patient, but this is the placebo response more often than not, and the symptoms typically come back.

This does not mean that having an operation is always unnecessary in the setting of IBS. Quite the contrary; if, for example, you experience a very severe pain in your upper abdomen that is quite different from your other IBS symptoms, this could be due to a problem such as gallstones. Before having an operation, however, you need to weigh the issues very carefully with your physician. Consider even seeking further opinions before having the procedure done, to be sure it is in your best interest. There is no such thing as a quick fix for an irritable bowel; you need to take control of your own health here. Remember another old adage: "if it ain't broke, don't fix it"—and even if it is broke a little, it don't necessarily need fixing, anyway. "Silent" gallstones (those not causing pain) just don't need to be taken out. One of the great principles of medical care is "first, cause no harm" (in Latin, *primum non nocere*). It is terribly easy (even for the best doctors) to initially misdiagnose and mislabel IBS.

HOW DO I JUDGE WHETHER A TREATMENT REALLY WORKS?

You need to take control of your body and the treatments that you receive for your symptoms. To do this, you must be informed, but in the modern world, information overload can be a real problem. Indeed, how do you obtain accurate information that will guide you? Even if you are an expert in the field of IBS, the amount of literature in this area remains enormous and grows every single day. You need tools to be able to sift through the mass of material out there, so that you can read what is really most useful and, with the assistance of your doctor and other relevant health care professionals, manage the problem. This is where evidence-based medicine can really help you. Guidelines are now available for deciding what you should read and how to judge the benefits objectively, regardless of the authors' opinions.

Evidence-Based Medicine

> "It has been said that man is a rationale animal. All my life
> I have been searching for evidence which could support this."
> (Bertrand Russell, 1872–1970)

It is critical to realize that many people believe that one treatment or another will work for IBS, but this does not mean it is true. The fact that something seems to work or ought to work doesn't mean it really does. As mentioned already, the placebo response can often explain any therapy that seems to work. However, what you really want to take is something that truly benefits you and that will do so for the longer term because IBS does not disappear by itself in many people.

In science, studies are done in the attempt to prove that any new therapy is worthless! The goal of a trial is to show, for example, that a new drug is no better than a placebo. However, if the new drug consistently shows itself to be better than a placebo in clinical trials, this is strong evidence that there is a real benefit from this new treatment. The same applies to any therapy in IBS; the therapy needs to be tested in proper trials before you can believe it really works. Many of the therapies touted on the Internet as being of value have never been subjected to any clinical trials; most are probably worthless, and some are probably even dangerous. Hence, the application of science here is critical. Using therapies that have successfully withstood standard attempts to demonstrate that they are useless is referred to as the *method of deduction* and remains the key tenet of the scientific method in medicine.

There have been many instances in which this approach has not been taken and medical experts have been completely misled. In the early 1960s, stomach freezing was used as a treatment of peptic ulcer disease. Surgeons were so impressed with this approach that thousands of freezing machines were purchased in the United States. However, when a proper randomized trial was done, it was found that gastric freezing was no better than no treatment of peptic ulcer at all, and there was indeed a small trend for those who underwent gastric freezing to have even worse results. Stomach freezing died a natural death after this trial. Peptic ulcers are now known to be most often caused by a specific bacterial infection (no wonder freezing was bound to fail). It is a pity that so many of the therapies touted for IBS have not themselves also died such a natural death.

When you read a scientific paper or newspaper or Internet report and are trying to find out whether the treatment really might work, there are some simple but key pieces of information you need to look at in order to work out whether you should believe what the author writes.[6,7] A strength of research published in scientific journals is that it all undergoes what is called peer review; this means that other experts in the field are asked to carefully read the paper and comment on its perceived accuracy and importance. However, many papers appear in the literature after this process with information that is just plain wrong. Some authors will even speculate further than the data allow, and this may not be picked up in the process. (A famous example of this relates to the controversy surrounding autism and vaccination in children. The authors speculated that a vaccine for measles caused childhood autism, which led to a huge outcry and fear that still echoes today.[8] Eventually, 10 of the 12 authors retracted the speculation—not the results—but the damage was done.) Papers are published primarily as a means of communication among scientists; publication of a paper doesn't mean that it's correct. Many papers report initial or preliminary results that could be exciting but are certainly not definitive (and often are just plain wrong).

So how can you work out what is really good science? Consider the following checklist when you look at a study on the Internet or in a book or in a magazine that reports a new treatment (see Chapter 9 for how to find such material).

- *Was the study a comparison of an active treatment with a placebo (a dummy treatment)?* Some trials for IBS compare an older active treatment with a newer active treatment, but most good trials include a placebo group. If there is no placebo, be really suspicious; the study won't be definitive! I won't believe the study establishes that a new therapy works unless there is a placebo group.
- *Were the patients included in the trial randomized to the active and comparison treatments?* The word "randomized" is absolutely critical here. It means that the authors used a system such as flipping a coin (or more likely, a computer program) to assign patients to the active treatment or to the placebo treatment. This is one of the central strengths of the current scientific method because randomization

means that people will not be assigned to one group or another because of a special characteristic or because investigators are putting the patients who are least sick on the new treatment. It is hoped that by randomization, the placebo and active treatment groups will be similar except for the fact that one received a specific type of therapy and the other did not. If you allow a nonrandomized method for assigning treatment, the investigators may consciously or unconsciously rig the trial in favor of the new therapy. Obviously, rigging a trial is not acceptable. So "randomization" is a critical term. If the trial looking at any new therapy is not randomized, ignore it and read something else.

- *Did the trial try to keep everyone blinded?* "Blinded" means that the investigators and the patients in the trial do not know which patients are receiving a placebo and which an active therapy. Of course, a record is kept elsewhere so that at the end of the trial, the investigators will know who got active therapy and who did not, but this information is kept concealed during the study. The idea here is that if you don't know what therapy someone is on, you will not be influenced by that knowledge when you are assessing how the treatment is working. You must remember that investigators desperately want to find treatments that work, to help their patients and to advance the field. The drug companies that sponsor clinical trials also desperately want their drugs to work (for their stockholders). Hence, if one actually knew who was on active therapy and who was not, this knowledge might subtly (and again, consciously or unconsciously) alter how one rates the benefit of the treatment. Not knowing makes the trial a better scientific study. If the trial is not blinded, then it is of limited value. *Double blind* means that both patients and investigators do not know what treatment is being given during the trial and is the standard term you will see in the medical literature.

It can be difficult or impossible to blind some treatments, however (such as hypnotherapy or acupuncture).

In the field of IBS, treatment that really works should have been subjected to a randomized, blinded, placebo-controlled trial. Even then, one trial is not sufficient; more that one trial showing the same result is much more convincing evidence for a real benefit. This is why the US Food and Drug Administration requires, for new drug approvals, that two large randomized double-blind placebo-controlled trials of active drug versus placebo be conducted to show that the new medication really is of benefit to IBS patients. Therapies that have not been subjected to randomized blinded placebo-controlled trials may work, but without the evidence for success, you should be very suspicious.

Weighing the Evidence

A number of randomized trials have tested whether fiber could be helpful in IBS, but the results have been very mixed, with both positive and negative studies in the medical literature. How can we judge whether fiber might really be helpful? The best way to do this is to undertake what is called a *meta-analysis*. Here, data from all of the clinical trials are looked at very carefully by a group of experts. The information from each trial is summarized in a similar way, and the results are then combined to determine whether the therapy could be of benefit overall. The probability that the therapy is better than the placebo can then be calculated. Indeed, software to do this has become available and makes the calculations relatively easy. The hardest part of a meta-analysis is actually extracting the right data from the trials so that they can be combined accurately. There is another problem: if all the trials are of poor quality (for example, too small in terms of the number of people tested), be concerned; in meta-analysis, rubbish in equals rubbish out.

High-quality meta-analyses are being published all the time now, and these are useful guides to finding the truth. One of the leading organizations conducting meta-analyses is the Cochrane Library (named after Archie Cochrane from England, who in 1979 called for the regular assembly of trials into a formal summary format). The Cochrane Library is used by researchers and scientists all over the world, and summaries of findings are published on the National Library of Medicine Web site, *PubMed* (see Chapter 9).

HOW ARE DRUG TREATMENTS THAT WORK IN IBS DEVELOPED?

"Half of the modern drugs could well be thrown out of the window, except that the birds might eat them." (Dr. Martin Henry Fischer)

Many different drugs for IBS treatment are on the market. Most of these came on the market before rigorous evidence was required to launch a treatment. In years gone by, drugs that appeared to be safe could be launched even if proof that they were better than a placebo (the "gold standard") was not available. This is no longer the case. New compounds that appear must be shown to have a benefit for symptoms over and above the important placebo response. Modern trials in IBS compare what is hoped to be an active compound with an inert (placebo) compound; the active compound must beat the inert compound in terms of showing a meaningful clinical benefit (in other words, make you better). Some trials compare a new treatment with an active drug that is known to be better than placebo, but there remains the need for placebo-controlled studies of IBS because no universally effective medicine yet exists.

Drug discovery and development is a fascinating process—and an expensive one. It typically takes about 12 years to dis-cover a drug and bring it to the patient. The cost to the drug company is $400 million (US) on average but can be much greater.[9] The process of drug discovery and development is highly regulated by the Food and Drug Administration (FDA) in the United States and by other regulatory bodies worldwide in order to ensure that only drugs that are safe and effective are finally available. Even so, new drugs can cause unexpected problems once in widespread use, leading to their withdrawal.

New drug research usually starts by studying how the body functions, both normally and abnormally. Diseases are complex and typically involve cascades of events at the cell level. It is important for researchers to understand what these actual events are at the most basic level so that they can identify a target at which to aim. This highly specialized work takes place in the laboratory and is done not only by some pharmaceutical companies but also at many top academic and government institutions. Sometimes there are existing molecules and compounds; hundreds and even thousands of these compounds can be tested before one of them will meet the requirements these scientists set. At other times, researchers will design a drug aimed at a specific target from scratch and synthesize it. A further approach is to test compounds made naturally by microscopic organisms. Antibiotics such as penicillin were discovered this way. Once a compound has been found to have an effect, modifications may be required to improve its action and profile. After this compound has been developed in the test tube, it needs to be tested in living animals. Animal testing is done in a regulated and (hopefully) humane manner, with as few animals as possible and with regard to their proper care. These tests will show if the potential drug will cause any obvious adverse events.

It is also important to understand how drugs are absorbed into the body, to which organ systems they distribute, how they are broken down (metabolized), and how they are eliminated from the body, as well as the rates at which these processes occur. These studies are called pharmacokinetic studies, and they are conducted early in the drug development process. Scientists can sometimes add other chemicals to drugs to change the absorption rate, either to help improve absorption or to prevent the drug from being broken down and excreted too soon. Such changes mean that more testing is required.

Testing of a new drug in humans begins with submission of information about the product to a formal regulatory agency and application for permission to begin administering the drug to healthy volunteers or to patients; in the United States, the formal regulatory agency is the FDA. In addition to receiving FDA approval, all clinical trial plans and informed-consent documents (which contain detailed information on the study for those who wish to participate) must be reviewed and approved by an institutional or independent review board (IRB). An IRB is a committee of physicians, community advocates, and others who try to ensure that a clinical trial is ethical and that the rights of the study's participants are protected.

Clinical testing in humans is done in three phases. Phase I clinical trials are designed to confirm the safety and tolerability of the drug in healthy human volunteers. Usually, this involves small numbers of healthy people who take the drug for a short period of time while being closely monitored. Sometimes these are people who volunteer for many studies for money; therefore, the results are really viewed as very preliminary.

Once safety and benefits are assessed and look acceptable, phase II clinical trial testing can begin. These studies determine the effectiveness of the drug in small numbers of patients with the disease or condition the drug is designed to treat. These studies can still involve several hundred patients and can take from 6 months to 3 years to complete. Testing is conducted with different doses to determine the best dose to use.

In addition, much more safety information is collected. Most phase II studies are randomized and blinded, which means that some patients receive a placebo or comparison drug instead of the test drug but that generally neither the patients nor their physicians know which drug the patients are receiving. This enables the results to be unbiased, and the advantage over a placebo or comparison drug can be determined.

A phase III trial commences when benefit seems highly likely and the dose range has been narrowed down. This phase consists of expanded testing for effectiveness and safety, usually in randomized and blinded studies involving several hundreds to thousands of patients, and typically lasts from 1 to 4 years.

Once these three phases of testing are complete, a new drug application is submitted to the regulatory agency (the FDA if in the United States). This application contains all the information about the drug, including reports of all laboratory, animal, and clinical studies. The benefits and safety profiles of the drug are carefully evaluated. This evaluation generally takes from 6 months to 2 years. After the regulatory agency approves the drug, pharmaceutical companies may conduct additional studies to expand the testing of the drug to a broader patient population, for example, or to determine the long-term effectiveness of the drug or provide more safety information.

As can be seen, the process is meticulous, lengthy, and expensive. Of every 5,000 new compounds identified during the discovery process, only about five are considered safe for human testing. After 3 to 6 years of further clinical evaluation, only one of these compounds is likely to be approved as a marketed drug. The research-based pharmaceutical industry invests about $12.6 billion (US) in research and development annually, and that investment has been doubling every 5 years. However, there are also justifiable criticisms that can be leveled at the industry, including the diversion of resources to develop "me too" drugs that bring in profits but do little (if anything) for patient care.

Problems still can occur once the drug reaches the market. Uncommon or rare side effects may not be detected until a drug is marketed and used by many thousands of people. So sometimes new treatments cause more harm than good. When I was in medical training, a wise physician once taught me to always avoid using new drugs, if alternatives are available, until there has been considerable experience with them. Unfortunately, there is no such thing as a completely safe drug, and the same goes for drugs used by alternative therapists (herbs are drugs!).

Drug names can be confusing. The generic name is what the drug is called; an example is omeprazole, which is the generic name of an acid pump blocker for heartburn. The trade name is the name the drug company uses to market a drug; for example, omeprazole is marketed as Prilosec and is now available over the counter. In the medical literature, the generic name, not the trade name, is usually used. When you are reading medical articles, this needs to be kept in mind.

PHARMACEUTICAL RESEARCH: BENEFITS AND DANGERS

The pharmaceutical industry has come under fire in recent times for unethical drug marketing practices and, in part, deservedly so. Although the development of new drugs is usually conducted ethically and carefully, once the drugs are on the market, advertising is permitted and can become very aggressive. This is directed at not only physicians but also the public, especially in the United States. Indeed, in most countries, TV advertising of pharmaceuticals is banned to protect the public, and this seems a remarkably sensible policy. This might have avoided, for example, the overprescription of Vioxx (rofecoxib), now linked to heart deaths. Pharmaceutical companies have undoubtedly raised sales and profits by their aggressive marketing strategies, but in some cases such sales have not led to improved health and may even have caused harm. However, the companies would also argue that they have assisted many people to become more aware of their health and to take action to receive treatment for a disease when they wouldn't necessarily have done so without being made aware by pharmaceutical TV advertising.

Unfortunately, by marketing to those who don't necessarily need or want their products, the pharmaceutical companies have left themselves open to public scrutiny and subsequent criticism for overemphasizing diseases that are not important or that do not need to be treated. IBS has been considered one of these diseases by some, as have other health problems such as heartburn or erectile dysfunctioin (impotence). However, IBS is very important to those whose lives are affected by the disease, so here at least the companies have a point.

The situation is complex. On occasion, pharmaceutical companies, who are responsible to their shareholders may employ what could be considered dubious marketing practices. A balance is needed between the public good and company profit making. There are now several sets of published guidelines to direct appropriate marketing practices by the pharmaceutical companies and to provide safeguards not only for the companies but also for medical professionals and the public with respect to the advertising and marketing of products.

Those in the medical profession who study drugs in clinical research have come under scrutiny because of their relationships with the pharmaceutical industry. The concern is that doctors who have any financial relationship with the industry may lose their public perspective or even choose to mislead the public. I, and most experts in the field of IBS, have regularly consulted with many pharmaceutical companies to assist with the development of new drugs (many of which never make it to market). For this professional advice, we often receive payments for the time we spend consulting (often on weekends and out of hours) or funding to undertake independent research studies. I believe that industry research funding is vital to supplement other sources (such as that from the government or donations) in order to be able to advance knowledge so that patients (who must come first) will benefit. Without this support, society would be much less able to develop or bring new drugs to market to better treat diseases for which we currently have no cure.

In the vast majority of cases, the financial recompense is modest, and there are specific requirements in place that ensure that doctors' relationships with the pharmaceutical industry, either as consultants or researchers, are appropriately monitored and disclosed. For example, at medical meetings doctors who present information on a disease or a drug are now expected to publicly list their relationships and activities with any relevant pharmaceutical company.

Overall, the companies need independent medical expertise and advice to make progress. Conversely, the researchers need new tools to study diseases, and the pharmaceutical industry often helps to develop these tools. Unfortunately, it is true that a small minority abuse the system. This is clearly not acceptable and must be dealt with appropriately. Sadly, as a result of this minority, some have called for an end to all or most relationships between independent medical experts in universities and the pharmaceutical industry, which is both unrealistic and reactionary. When conducted ethically and openly, I believe that a working partnership between the pharmaceutical industry and the available independent medical expertise is synergistic, indeed essential. We need such interactions in order to continue to advance our understanding of IBS and similar diseases, to the benefit of all sufferers.

Take-Home Messages

- Medical trials try to prove that something doesn't work! This is the "scientific method." (Of course, trials are done in the hope that the treatment will beat the placebo and thus be shown to be helpful.)
- Placebos (dummy treatments) can help; however, their benefit may not last.
- IBS treatments that have not been compared with a placebo are not of any established benefit, no matter how many testimonials are quoted.
- Use evidence-based medicine to help you decide if a treatment really does work.

CHAPTER 5

DIET AND EXERCISE: KEY HELPERS IN THE BATTLE

"Everything from oatmeal and fruit to a regular dinner causes pain and bloating. I rarely feel motivated to exercise or have the energy. I dread every bowel movement."

"I was fearful of eating out, and when I did, I took my own food—my friends were very kind about it."

"My diet has given me back my life, and I would be very happy if it could help anyone else."

"I gave the elimination diet my best try. To my immense relief, the pain due to bloating ceased, and I began to feel a lot better. It has taken me 5 years to work out my own regimen for comfort."

HOW DO I NORMALLY DIGEST FOOD?

You drink and eat so that carbohydrates, protein, and fat, as well as vitamins and minerals, can enter your body and be used for fuel or essential chemical reactions. To make use of ingested food substances, they need to be broken down into small units that can then be absorbed. A number of different enzymes attack food substances to help break them down. Enzymes are usually proteins that catalyze chemical reactions to break down specific food substances. Salivary gland enzymes break down carbohydrates and fats; enzymes from the pancreas break down carbohydrates, proteins, and fats. Once substances have been broken down in the small bowel, they next pass through the lining of the bowel and into the bloodstream. This occurs by a number of different processes and depends on the particular food substance. Most digestion does not occur in the stomach but in the small bowel.

Understanding these processes can help you plan how best to use diet to treat irritable bowel syndrome (IBS).

Carbohydrate Absorption

Starches consist of a combination of sugar (glucose) molecules that are digested in the small bowel. Examples include milk sugar (lactose) and table sugar (sucrose). Saliva contains an enzyme called amylase that will break down starch initially. In the small bowel, amylase released from the pancreas will break down the rest of the starch. Additional digestion of the derivatives of starch are broken down by enzymes along the lining of the small bowel. Lactase, one of these enzymes in the bowel, breaks down lactose into glucose and galactose. In people who are *lactase deficient*, the lactose is not broken down, and it drags out water from the cells into the bowel itself. This can lead to diarrhea with bloating and excess gas.

About 1 in 6 people in the United States who are descended from Europeans will have a problem with drinking milk because they are lactase deficient. The majority of black, Asian, and Native Americans will be lactase deficient in adulthood. People with lactase deficiency are sometimes misdiagnosed as having IBS.

Bacteria exist in huge amounts in the colon and can further break down carbohydrates that are not absorbed higher up in the small bowel. Their actions lead to the production of excess gas (with carbon dioxide and oxygen). Some bacteria in the bowel ("stink bugs") eat hydrogen, leading to the release of methane gas or sulfur-containing gases. This can lead to a very distinct awful odor you may smell after a bowel movement.

Protein Absorption

In the stomach, protein digestion begins with the breakdown of the linkages across the protein products (peptides) by the enzyme pepsin that is released in the stomach. Pepsins are activated in an acid environment, and this occurs in the stomach because it secretes hydrochloric acid (unless you are taking a strong acid suppressing medicine or have a stomach disease). The protein products (peptides) are further digested in the small intestine because of the breakdown by enzymes secreted by the pancreas, in particular, trypsin and the chymotrypsins. However, the small bowel can still handle this process without difficulty if the stomach is removed completely. Final digestion occurs along the lining of the small bowel and in the small bowel cells themselves.

Fat Absorption

Lipase is an important enzyme that breaks down fats. A very small amount of this lipase comes from the tongue and is activated in the stomach. However, almost all fat digestion normally occurs because of the secretion of lipase from the pancreas into the small bowel. Lipase breaks down fat into free fatty acids. Bile is also secreted into the small bowel from the gallbladder and activates a specific lipase that helps break down cholesterol. The fat and bile salts, when they are in high concentration in the small bowel, spontaneously group together to form circular structures called micelles. The micelles take up fat and transport it to the small-bowel wall, where the fat can be presented and absorbed by the cells lining the small intestine. The bile salts then travel down the small bowel alone.

The bile salts are then taken up (reabsorbed) by the end of the small bowel (called the terminal ileum). However, some bile salts can spill over into the colon, causing diarrhea as they stimulate the colon cells to squirt out water. Bile salts can be more likely to spill over if the gallbladder has been removed, because the gallbladder's job is to hold onto bile and release it only with a meal. With no gallbladder, bile is continuously released into the small bowel from the liver. These bile salts can be "mopped up" by certain drugs, which can ease the diarrhea in some people with IBS.

In the absence of the enzyme lipase, diarrhea occurs and the stool is full of fat. In this case, the stool is typically white, large in volume, and very difficult to flush away. It is also very smelly, and you may see oil droplets in the toilet bowl; this is called steatorrhea. The weight-loss drug orlistat (Xenical) blocks lipase so that fat cannot be absorbed properly; this is why people taking this drug may get diarrhea, pass lots of awful gas, and have fatty stools (which means some people just don't tolerate this weight-loss drug for long).

Water and Electrolytes

The gastrointestinal tract secretes a large amount of fluid. About 7 L (1.8 gallons) of this fluid comes from the lining of the small bowel and its glands (1 liter = ¼ gallon). In addition, you normally drink about 2 L (about ½ gallon) of fluid per day. On the other hand, you lose only about 200 mL of fluid (⅒ gallon) through the bowel motions; 98% is typically reabsorbed in the small bowel and colon. The presence of glucose helps the absorption of salt and water in the small bowel. This is why treatment with salt and water (electrolyte solutions) is given when traveler's diarrhea is severe and is leading to dehydration. On the other hand, substances that leach out water and salt from the bowel wall will cause diarrhea (for example, milk of magnesia is a laxative that works in this way).

The colon (also called the large intestine because it is bigger in diameter) absorbs 90% of the fluid that reaches it normally, so there is about 200 mL of water in the stool of a healthy person. Stool also contains other inorganic materials as well as bacteria and undigested plant fibers. Because much of the stool is composed of normal secretions from the bowel, you will still pass some stool in health even if you starve yourself. However, if you eat nothing, you will usually become constipated (as one of my surgical colleagues who specializes in constipation surgery tells his patients, "if you don't eat, you won't poop!"). People with anorexia nervosa, an eating disorder, often are constipated. The brown color of stool is due to pigmentation from the bile salts broken down by bacteria in the large bowel (this is also why it normally smells!).

It takes about 4 hours for a meal to go from the stomach to the first part of the colon. At the end of the small bowel, there is a valve (called the ileocecal valve) that squeezes shut if the pressure in the colon increases but opens if the pressure at the end of the small bowel goes up. This is to prevent surging of contents from the colon back into the small bowel. When the peristaltic wave reaches the end of the small bowel, the ileocecal valve briefly opens (relaxes) and allows some of the material to squirt into the colon.

The reflex pathway between the stomach and the colon is called the gastrocolic reflex. As food starts to leave the stomach, the pressure on material around the valve at the end of the small bowel increases, and the right side of the colon starts to relax, probably because the vagus nerve becomes stimulated from the stomach, signaling the brain and then the colon.

Your colon goes to sleep when you do; when you get up in the morning and have breakfast, you will often feel the urge to go to the toilet soon afterwards (the "breakfast rush"). This is the gastrocolic response in action! Some people with IBS possibly have an exaggerated gastrocolonic response, which might explain why their symptoms are worse in the morning (although this is somewhat speculative).

Material is moved through the colon by contraction of muscle over large areas. These are called high-amplitude propagated contractions, and they promote the movement of material from one portion of the colon toward the end (anus). There are other contractions in the colon that mix the contents, helping absorption.

In a healthy person, when the rectum becomes swollen (distended) with stool, this stimulates contraction of the muscle reflexly and signals the desire to go to the toilet (part of the brain is switched on by the swelling in the rectum). When the rectum becomes distended, the muscle around the rectum that normally prevents the leakage of stool (the anal sphincter) relaxes. You can voluntarily relax the part of the anal sphincter that is called the external sphincter. Relaxing this muscle is important in helping normal defecation. Tensing the abdominal-wall muscles (straining) also will help empty the rectum. One can block defecation by contracting the external anal sphincter even though one has the urge to go. You can do this now or anytime: tell yourself to squeeze your anus shut; this is the external anal sphincter in action. The internal anal sphincter, on the other hand, is not under voluntary control. Thus, many factors can affect bowel function. For example, you can learn (unconsciously) to squeeze shut the external anal sphincter when it should be being relaxed, which can contribute to worsening constipation in some people. Thankfully, this can be "unlearned" with the help of biofeedback (page 109), which can substantially improve constipation.

DIETARY FIBER

Humans are unable to digest a number of vegetable products, including cellulose and other plant carbohydrates. "Fiber" refers to any ingested food that will reach the large bowel (large intestine or colon) without being affected by the digestive process. (Strictly speaking, "fiber" refers to carbohydrates we can't digest, but there are other undigestible materials that are fiberlike.) Fiber has a large number of different components, including cellulose, hemicellulose, lignin, and pectin. Bowel movements are less frequent if there is a smaller amount of dietary fiber in a person's diet than there should be. Unfortunately, the American diet is traditionally low in fiber;

this is further aggravated by the fast-food industry, which serves generally low-fiber diets high in carbohydrates and fats.

Should I Change the Fiber in My Diet, and If So, How?

"The second day of a diet is always easier than the first. By the second day you're off it." (Jackie Gleason, 1916-1987)

People with IBS may benefit from increasing the fiber in their diets. This means increasing the roughage or bulk that is eaten. Plant foods that cannot be digested or absorbed by the human body increase stool bulk (hence they are called bulking agents). Eating lots of fiber can have all sorts of potential health benefits. Fiber can make the stools soft if they have been hard, because the undigested material leaches out water from the large bowel into the stool itself. On the other hand, people with loose stools sometimes find that fiber helps firm up the stools, although this is variable.

Fiber helps reduce the amount of pressure that the bowel needs to exert to move its contents, which can help the pain, at least in some people although, sadly, this benefit is not very evident from clinical trials.[1,2] There is some evidence that high-fiber diets reduce colon cancer and heart disease, but it is not conclusive.

In terms of taking in more fiber, a trick that helps many people with IBS is this; make sure that you only gradually change the amount of fiber in your diet. A sudden increase in dietary fiber will, more likely than not, make you feel bloated and gassy. However, if you slowly increase the amount of fiber in the diet, the increase is usually much better tolerated and often will not cause more problems but may actually be helpful.

Types of Fiber

It is important to realize that there are two different types of dietary fiber and that they vary very much in the diet.

Insoluble fiber is present in wheat bran, whole grains, and some vegetables. Soluble fiber is present in dried beans and peas, oats, and some fruits and vegetables. Soluble fiber can help reduce cholesterol and blood sugar levels, which can be useful for people who suffer with high cholesterol levels or diabetes. Soluble and insoluble fiber both seem to be effective in helping people with constipation. Soluble fiber supplements (but not insoluble fiber) have been shown to be of benefit to IBS patients in clinical trials.[2]

How Can I Best Increase Dietary Fiber in My Diet?

Changing your diet can be helpful. The average American diet has about half the amount of fiber needed for the best of health. Therefore, even if you have no bowel symptoms, increasing dietary fiber, if you can tolerate it, may be useful. For people with IBS, increasing fiber should be tried as the first line of treatment of the condition. However, it is important to do this in a sensible way as eating more fiber may otherwise make one's symptoms worse.

It is generally recommended that people eat 20 to 30 g of fiber a day, about twice the normal American diet's fiber content. Eating more than 50 g of fiber a day just doesn't help, so don't try to eat too much. The cheapest way to increase the fiber is to have a well-balanced diet whereby you are eating more whole-grain breads and cereals, more vegetables and fruits, and more dried beans and peas (if this doesn't make you too gassy). It is also sensible to eat regularly scheduled meals with some increased fiber-enriched foods with every meal. This is most likely to promote healthy bowel function throughout the day, which is what you need when you have IBS.

Start off by increasing the fiber very slowly. If you eat too much fiber too quickly when your body is not used to it, you are more likely to experience bloating and gas. So consider introducing a small amount of high-fiber foods with each meal and increasing this amount every week until you reach adequate levels of fiber every day.

Table 5-1 will help you develop a fiber-containing diet that can assist you. Try to add no more than an additional 3 g of fiber daily each week. It will take about a month to get up to a total of 25 to 30 g of fiber per day if you are eating a normal diet now (which contains about 15g). You can work out the amount of fiber in most foods if you read the labels carefully.

An inexpensive way to add fiber to hot or cold cereal is to sprinkle on one tablespoon of unprocessed wheat bran. You can add two teaspoons the following week and three tablespoons in the third week if you are tolerating the increased bulk without problems. Unfortunately, the most recent evidence is that wheat bran does not help many IBS symptoms, but it can aid constipation.[2]

You can also add bran cereal or unprocessed wheat bran to a whole series of other foods, including breads and muffins, cookies and cakes, and meatloaf and casseroles. You can replace a cup of white flour with ⅞ cup of coarsely ground wheat flour or 1 cup of finely milled wheat flour. Try having soups, salads, or main dishes that contain dried peas or beans, lentils, or whole grains, but you will have to experiment here to get the best flavor as well as the best-tolerated combination. Try eating brown rice or whole wheat pasta as either side dishes or in your soups or casseroles. Add raw vegetables if you like them. Eat plenty of dried fruit. Replace potato chips and candy with popcorn. Don't eat so many cakes or cookies, but try eating desserts with fruit or bran muffins.

When you are eating more fiber, it is important to drink enough fluid. Fiber absorbs more liquid in your large bowel; therefore, you need to drink enough fluid, or you may aggravate rather than relieve the symptoms of constipation (although the evidence here is weak). It is generally recom-

Table 5-1:   Fiber Content of Various Foods

2–3 g fiber per serving

Grain products*

Barley, cooked

Bran muffin

Bread or roll, 100% whole wheat

Bulgur, cooked

Cheerios, 1 cup

Crispbread, whole grain
(eg, Ry Krisp), 2 pieces

Granola

Grape-Nuts Flakes, 1 cup

Life, 1 cup

Muesli

Oat bran cereal, cooked

Oatmeal, cooked

Popcorn, 2–3 cups

Wheat bran, 2 tbsp

Hot wheat cereal (eg, Ralston,
Maltex, Wheatena)

Wheat flakes (eg, Wheaties, Total),
1 cup

Wheat germ, 2 tbsp

Whole wheat spaghetti or macaroni,
cooked

Vegetables and fruits†

Artichokes

Bamboo shoots

Beets

Broccoli

Brussels sprouts

Carrots

Cauliflower

Corn

Cucumber, large

Green beans

Greens

Kohlrabi

Parsnips

Peas, green

Potato

Rutabaga

Spinach

Squash, winter (eg, butternut,
buttercup)

Sweet potato

Tomato, large

Tomato sauce or paste

Wax beans

Apple

Apricots, fresh, 4–5

Banana

Blueberries

Cherries

Dried fruit, ¼ cup

Figs, canned

Figs, fresh, 2

Kiwi

Mango

Nectarine

Orange

Papaya

Prunes, cooked or canned

Nuts, ¼ cup

Peanut butter, 2 tbsp

Snack seed kernels, ¼ cup

Table 5-1: Fiber Content of Various Foods (continued)

4–6 g fiber per serving

Grain products★

    Bran flakes, 1 cup

    Wheat Chex or Multi-Bran Chex, 1 cup

    Corn Bran, 1 cup

    Grape-Nuts ½ cup

    Raisin Bran, 1 cup

    Shredded wheat cereal, 1 cup bite-sized or 2 biscuits

Vegetables and fruits†

    Avocado

    Baked beans

    Dried beans (eg, navy, pinto, kidney, lima, soy), cooked or canned

    Lentils, cooked

    Dried peas, cooked

    Pumpkin

    Vegetable protein burger

    Blackberries

    Figs, dried, ¼ cup

    Pear

    Raspberries

    Strawberries

> 6 g fiber per serving

    Bran cereal (eg, All-Bran, Fiber One, 100% Bran, Bran Buds), ½ cup

---

★One serving of a grain product is 1/2 cup or 1 average piece unless otherwise specified.

†One serving of a vegetable or fruit is 1/2 cup cooked, 1 cup raw, or 1 average piece unless otherwise specified.

mended that you drink 8 to 10 or more 8 oz glasses of non-caffeinated liquid each day. Caffeine-containing drinks are dehydrating, unfortunately. Water is excellent!

Remember that you don't just need to eat fiber; you must have a balanced diet. Fish, poultry, and meat don't have fiber but have other important nutrients, including protein, which you must get from somewhere. On the other hand, unfortunately, desserts and sweets (as well as fats) have lots of extra calories but little or no fiber, so avoid these treats as much as you can stand.

I Can't Stand Increasing the Fiber in My Diet Naturally, so What about Fiber Supplements?

"I supplement each meal with one-half tablespoon of fiber supplement to provide some roughage and avoid constipation."

The experts often say that fiber supplements have few advantages, aside from convenience, over increasing the fiber content of your diet naturally. In my experience, however, many people prefer this approach. Moreover, clinical trials with fiber supplements (also called bulking agents) have shown that some of them are better than placebo![2] So it is reasonable to try them, but remember that it will also cost you more. Fiber supplements work best if you have more constipation than diarrhea. Still, they can help firm up loose stools in some people.

There are lots of different fiber supplements on the market and little to choose between them. Go and look in your pharmacy and read the labels. Some of the fiber products that you will find there include Metamucil, Perdiem Fiber, and Konsyl (these contain psyllium); FiberCon (contains calcium polycarbophil); and Citrucel (contains methylcellulose). They may come in powder, biscuit, tablet, wafer, or toasted granule form, but the actual presentation of the fiber probably makes little difference. When you read the label, you will find that 1 teaspoon of most of the powdered fiber supplements has about 3 to 6 g of fiber (see Chapter 7). Therefore, aim to eventually take about three doses a day (approximately 10–15 g of fiber) if you are supplementing a normal American diet although some people will need only 1 or 2 doses daily. Premeasured packets and tablets are more costly but add convenience. Start slow, and build up the dose you take very gradually (initially no more than one-half to one dose daily, and increase the amount every 1 to 2 weeks only until you are taking two to three doses in total).

Many fiber supplements are psyllium based. Psyllium is also in a few cereal products such as Kellogg's Bran Buds ready to eat. The best evidence for a benefit of fiber supplements in IBS is for psyllium products; psyllium is better than placebo for helping the symptoms of IBS.[2] Psyllium comes from a soluble grain. When you mix psyllium with a liquid, drink it right away; otherwise, it will gel and become much less pleasant to drink.

Remember to use an unsweetened powder, which is calorie free, if weight loss is another benefit you are seeking or if you are diabetic. Examples include sugar-free Metamucil, Fiberall, and Konsyl, all of which have no added sugar. If you do use a fiber drink, it may make you feel full before a meal and can help you lose weight (if you desire to, of course). On the other hand, if you happen to be underweight, consider taking your fiber supplement drink after a meal rather than before, and avoid calorie-free products. Some of the products are low in sodium or sodium free, but this varies, so do look at the label on the product if this is an issue for you (eg, if you have high blood pressure). Remember too that psyllium can have side effects (see page 135). For example, allergies have been reported, and although these are rare, they do occur. Overall, psyllium is one of the safest treatments we have for IBS and can be taken by most people who tolerate it regularly over the long term.

I HAVE EXCESS GAS; CAN DIET HELP?

Swallowing air and producing gas in the bowel is normal. However, some people have a tendency to swallow more air as they eat. Others seem to produce more gas in their bowels. This may be related partly to the different compositions of the bacterial colonies present in the bowel. Indeed, a normal colon contains an enormous mass of bacteria. The colon is sterile at birth, but very soon after, the entire bowel acquires billions of bugs of different species. Most live in the colon, but there are smaller numbers in the small bowel in health (acid from the stomach kills most of the bacteria, so it is usually clean). These bacteria act like a factory, and gas is one of their by-products.

A number of foods can be linked to increasing the production of gas in the bowel. However, the foods that do this vary in their effect from person to person, and therefore it takes a lot of trial and error to find the foods that you

Table 5-2:   Foods That May Be Gas Forming

Legumes and vegetables

Baked beans	Kohlrabi
Dried beans	Lentils
Lima beans	Onions
Broccoli	Dried peas
Brussels sprouts	Radishes
Cabbage	Rutabagas
Cauliflower	Sauerkraut
Cucumbers	

Fruits and fruit juices (excessive amounts)

Prunes	Prune juice
Apples	Apple juice
Raisins	Grape juice
Bananas	

Grain products

Bran

Dairy products

Milk	
Cream	Ice cream
	Ice milk

should avoid. Table 5-2 lists some common foods that can cause gas.

Baked beans are a typical example of gas-producing foods, and some people eat these and take great pleasure in expelling gas through the mouth after a meal or later from the other end. However, people with gas trouble don't want to deal with this issue, so cutting out beans and the other legumes and vegetables that are particularly gas forming can be helpful. Fruits and fruit juices (especially prunes, prune juice, grape juice, and apple juice) can also produce a lot of gas. All high-fiber products produce more gas, and this can be a real problem for those who are trying to increase the fiber in their diets. A list of less-gassy fiber-containing foods appears in Table 5-3.

Table 5-3: Fiber-Containing Foods That Are Less Gas Forming

Fruits	Vegetables	Grain Products
Apricots, fresh	Asparagus	Barley
Berries	Beans, green or wax	Bread, whole wheat
Nectarines	Beets	Cereals, whole grain, such as:
Oranges, fresh	Carrots	Cheerios, Granola
Peaches, fresh	Corn	Oat Squares, Ralston
Pears	Greens	Grape-nuts, Maltex
Pineapple	Okra	Shredded Wheat, Total
Plums, fresh	Peas, green	Mini-Wheats, muesli
	Potatoes (with skin)	Muslix
	Spinach	Wheat Chex, Wheaties
	Sweet potatoes	Wheatena, Nutri-Grain
	Pumpkin	Flat breads and crispbreads,
	Tomatoes	whole grain, such as:
	Winter squash	Kavli, Wasa
		Pasta, whole wheat
		Popcorn
		Rice, brown or wild
		Ry Krisp

Again, it must be emphasized that each individual person will vary in this respect. Dairy products such as milk, ice cream, ice milk, and cream can produce a feeling of excess gas, particularly if there is any lactose intolerance. However, even if there is no lactose intolerance, these products can sometimes seem to be associated with feelings of less gas when they are eliminated from the diet. Most people with lactose intolerance can have at least ½ cup of a dairy product at a time, without any major problems. Furthermore, yogurt, cheese, and cottage cheese usually don't cause any problems, even if there is a milk or cream intolerance.

Artificial sweeteners in sugar-free gum, diet candy, and diet drinks can also cause problems. Some people consume a lot of diet products every day. I've had patients who drink 6 to 12 cans of Diet Coke or Diet Pepsi a day (the caffeine load can be troublesome). If the artificial sweetener is sorbitol or mannitol, problems can occur because the sweetener is not absorbed and draws out fluid into the bowel. Other artificial sweeteners, such as aspartame (e.g. in Diet Coke or Pepsi) or saccharin (contained in Tab, for example), tend not to cause the same problem of excess gas, diarrhea, and bloating.

Another food group that you should particularly think about in terms of gas problems are high-fat foods. Fried foods, rich sauces and gravies, fatty meat, and rich pastries can contain lots of fat. Indeed, the American diet is full of fat. Items sold by fast-food outlets often have an extremely high fat content that one may not really appreciate (particularly for those who seek low carbs in their weight-losing diet, high fat may be substituted for taste). However, excess fat can cause gas and feelings of bloating in some people. High-fat foods slow stomach emptying and can also worsen feelings of indigestion and heartburn for those who also have this problem.

Reducing Belching and Air Swallowing

If you have a problem with burping (belching) repeatedly, it is likely that you are swallowing air. This is because you just cannot make enough air in the stomach or small bowel to belch repeatedly, even if you wanted to. The only way to do this is to swallow the air and then belch it back up. This can be quite unconscious, so you don't realize that excess air is being swallowed.

Knowing that you may be doing this helps, as does consciously trying not to swallow air. Remaining in the upright position after eating can help relieve this gas problem. It is important to avoid frequent or repetitive swallowing of air when you eat. Eating slowly rather than eating fast can help. Foods such as whipped creams and carbonated drinks contain lots of air, so stopping the use of these often is useful too. Don't gulp down your food or frequently sip through a straw, and avoid drawing on cigarettes or cigars or pipes. If you are a smoker, giving up smoking can help reduce air swallowing. In fact, smoking has so many health risks, you would be doing yourself a real favor, and this may eventually save your life; start by stopping right now and stick to your resolution (and see your physican for help if you can't stop). Avoid chewing gum and chewing tobacco. Not sucking on hard candies can reduce the amount of air that you swallow. Ill-fitting dentures can sometimes cause a problem leading to increased air swallowing; if you have this difficulty, see your dentist.

Some people swallow air as part of a nervous habit. Excess belching sometimes occurs when one is under particular stress; reducing stress can be helpful here. It may take a series of sessions with an experienced psychologist to learn how to reduce or abolish such a habit, and this is worth considering in difficult cases. Finally, regular exercise seems to help some people with this problem although the reasons (aside from stress reduction) are not obvious, and there have been no randomized trials. Treating constipation also sometimes helps reduce excess gas, perhaps because constipation triggers the stomach to empty more slowly.

Reducing Flatus

Flatus (gas being expelled through the anus) can be an awful problem for some people. Normally, we all expel gas about 13 times a day (less than 20 times is normal); this was learned by counting flatus episodes in the laboratory in health volunteers (a memorable experiment). Remember though, that whereas you may be aware of passing gas, many around you truly will not notice.

A special diet may help excess flatus. Flatus-producing foods include beans, brussels sprouts, onions, celery, carrots, raisins, bananas, wheat germ, and fermentable fiber, and pork can produce very smelly gases occasionally. Avoid these, then! Beano (a commercial product containing α-galactosidase, a sugar-digesting enzyme) is available over the counter; it can reduce the production of gas from eating baked beans. Use 3 to 8 drops on your food. Beano cannot be added to food being cooked because the enzyme is broken down by heat. You should not use Beano if you have the very rare disease galactosemia.

Try a "low-flatus" diet; this includes meat, fowl, fish, and eggs. Other low-flatus foods are gluten-free bread, rice bread, and rice; some vegetables, such as lettuce and tomatoes; and some fruits, such as cherries and grapes. If the diet works, introduce each potential "high-flatus" food that you have excluded every week and see if the gas returns; if it does, continue to avoid that food, but reintroduce another food product, and so on until you find the right mix. See a dietician for help if you are having trouble.

Products that contain chlorophyll (such as Derifil or Nullo) can reduce the odor from flatus. A charcoal cushion that you can buy can also be used for this purpose.

WHAT IS LACTOSE INTOLERANCE (LACTASE DEFICIENCY)?

If you experience bloating or cramping abdominal pain, excessive gas, or diarrhea, these symptoms could be explained by the fact that you are lactose intolerant. Lactase, an enzyme in the intestine, is essential for the body to be able to break down lactose, a sugar in milk products. The problem is that if lactase is no longer present in the body, then undigested lactose remains in the small-bowel and water is dragged into it. This leads to excessive frothy liquid being present in the bowel and to symptoms.

Most people in the world become lactase deficient naturally. Black and Hispanic people typically will be lactase deficient by the time they are adults. However, even if you are lactase deficient, you still can tolerate some lactose; a half cup of milk or a high-lactose food at any one time will not usually cause any problems. However, if you drink more than a cup of milk in this situation, you may get symptoms as the normal small bowel mechanisms in those without lactase are overwhelmed. For this reason, people with lactase deficiency can take small amounts of lactose throughout the day, and this will usually be tolerated well. It is also better if the lactose-containing food is taken with other foods at the same time as this combination tends to be better tolerated. So, if you are lactase deficient, you don't have to miss out on your ice cream treat or milk shake as long as you don't take in too much at a time.

Yogurt is better tolerated than other milk products because it contains good bacteria that digest part of the lactose anyway. Yogurt with an active culture is usually the best tolerated, but frozen yogurt may also be quite acceptable to your bowel. A list of lactose-free and low-lactose foods is summarized in Table 5-4. Remember, however, that almost

Table 5-4: Lactose-Free and Low-Lactose Food

Lactose free (may be used as desired)

Bread made without milk, dry milk solids, or whey (eg, Italian bread)
Broth-based soups
Cereals and crackers
Nondairy creamers
Desserts made without milk, dry milk solids, or whey
Fruits and vegetables
Plain meat, fish, poultry, and peanut butter
Special foods, such as cottage cheese, that are labeled "lactose-free"

Low lactose (tolerated by most people)

Aged and processed cheeses (eg, aged cheddar or Swiss, processed American)
Breads containing milk, dry milk solids, or whey
Butter and margarine
Commercially prepared foods containing dry milk solids or whey
Milk treated with lactase enzyme★
Sherbet

★Dairy Ease or Lactaid enzyme can be purchased in liquid or tablet form and can aid in the digestion of milk and milk products (follow the directions on the package).

nobody needs to be on a completely lactose-free diet, even if they have lactase deficiency.

You can be tested for lactose intolerance in a number of different ways by your doctor. A blood test can be done after you have a lactose load, to see if you have a problem with absorbing lactose. Another way is to have a breath test in which you eat a lactose load and the breath is tested for the amount of hydrogen present, which indicates whether or not you have absorbed the lactose (lactose is broken down by colon bacteria with the release of hydrogen if it is not well absorbed). A physician can also obtain a small amount of tissue from the small bowel by taking off a piece through an endoscope; this is totally painless because there are no pain fibers in the bowel lining. The specimen can be tested for the presence of enzymes, including lactase, but this is expensive.

Lots of people with IBS have lactase deficiency, but if your symptoms persist despite your following a low-lactose diet for 2 weeks, this almost certainly means that lactase deficiency is not the cause of your symptoms, and you can go back to eating a sensible diet that includes some lactose. A list of high-lactose foods to avoid if you are intolerant of lactose is shown in Table 5-5. If you are lactase deficient and are getting symptoms from eating high-lactose foods, lactase can be bought in tablet or liquid form (eg, Lactaid, Dairy Ease). The tablets can be chewed before eating lactose products, or the liquid can be added to milk.

FOOD INTOLERANCE AND FOOD ALLERGY

"'Just psychosomatic,' say most of the textbooks. The patient projects his conflicts onto his digestive system. Undeterred, I sought more information. As a biologist, I knew the technique of poring through recent medical articles listed in Index Medicus, MEDLINE, and Science Citation Index. Finally, eureka! One article stood out like a speck of gold in the bottom of a miner's pan. It suggested IBS can be caused by food intolerance and listed the most common foods that give problems. They are cheese, onions, milk, wheat, chocolate, butter, yogurt, coffee, eggs, nuts, rye, potatoes, barley, oats, and corn. Other books and papers echoed these findings and emphasized that more cereals, fatty foods, and too much fiber may intensify IBS symptoms. Beef can be a problem, too. Since there is no test for food intolerance, one has to learn what to avoid by use of an elimination diet and a food diary."

"Could food allergy be my problem?" Many patients believe it is, but food allergy causing IBS is very rare. Occasionally, people will experience swelling around the mouth or even more serious problems when they eat a food to which they are allergic. Peanut allergy is a classic example, which is why

Table 5-5: High-Lactose Foods to Consider Avoiding if You Have True Lactose Intolerance and Symptoms

Food	Serving Size
Cheese food or spread★	2 oz
Cottage cheese	¾ cup
Dry cottage cheese	1 cup
Ricotta cheese	¾ cup
Dry milk (whole, nonfat, buttermilk)	2 tbsp
Evaporated milk	¼ cup
Half-and-half	½ cup
Ice cream, ice milk	¾ cup
Milk (whole, skim, 1%, 2%, chocolate, buttermilk)	½ cup
Chip dip, potato topping	½ cup
Sour cream	½ cup
Sweet acidophilus milk	½ cup
Sweetened condensed milk	3 tbsp
White sauce	½ cup

★Labeled as such; lactose content is higher than that of aged and processed cheese because whey powder and/or dry milk solids are included.

many airlines now serve only those awful pretzels in coach class (as well, it probably saves them big money). However, almost everyone with IBS does not have true food allergy, and testing for food allergy is almost always unhelpful. Some people have tests done anyway, and positive reactions will be found, but if the foods are eliminated, the symptoms usually don't disappear (or if they do, it's that placebo response again). Hence, these food allergy test results are really false positives, a very common problem.

On the other hand, there is some evidence that certain foods eaten by people with IBS cause specific problems although the mechanism of this remains largely unclear. This situation is called food intolerance.[3] A large number of different foods have been implicated here, but the evidence for eliminating them has been mixed (Figure 5-1). However, a key clinical trial has suggested that food intolerance may be more important in some people with IBS than has been thought.[3] In this study, the investigators tested whether antibodies to foods (immunoglobulin G antibodies, to be exact, developed by York Test Laboratories Ltd, York, UK) were present in the blood. On the basis of this blood test, they then randomly (by chance, using a computer) allocated 150 people to either (1) a diet in which foods with positive antibodies were removed or (2) a "sham diet" where only foods where no antibodies were found to be positive on the blood test were removed. The investigators and the patients did not know which group the patients were in (all were "blinded"). People on the sham diet continued to eat the foods to which they had positive antibodies although other foods were removed so that no one knew whether or not they had received an active intervention. (Of course, a code was available to look at once the study ended, to "unblind" the investigators). The results were fascinating: those who were in the active-treatment group and whose diet contained none of the foods to which

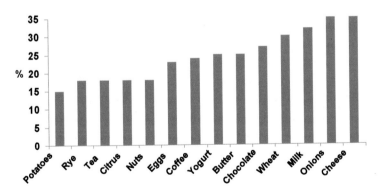

Figure 5-1: Food intolerance: common food items incriminated by patients with irritable bowel syndrome (*n* = 189). Adapted and printed with permission from Nanda R, James R, Smith H, et al. Food intolerance and the irritable bowel syndrome. Gut 1989;30:1099–104.

they had antibodies definitely did better than the group on the sham diet. The most commonly implicated foods were milk, cheese, eggs, peas and beans, various nuts, shellfish, chicken, and wheat-containing products. These results remain to be confirmed, but they suggest that some people with IBS who do not respond to the usual dietary recommendations as discussed above might still respond to the elimination of certain foods from their diets. However, one needs to be very careful; a number of different foods will upset people with IBS, and this is variable. However, this does not mean that they are food intolerant since increased bowel sensitivity is a major abnormality in the majority of people with IBS. Unfortunately, the blood test used in the trial discussed above is not yet widely available commercially and has not been sufficiently tested to be recommended.

Testing for food intolerance can also be done with the introduction of a very bland diet and then the slow reintroduction of a number of different foods to see whether or not these induce symptoms, but the process is very laborious and expensive. However, if you are particularly troubled with IBS and standard treatments have failed, it would be worth considering looking into food intolerance with the help of your physician and an expert dietician.

HOW CAN THE BOWELS BE MADE REGULAR?

Obsession with the bowels is not a recent phenomenon. There is a wonderful review of the subject in the *British Medical Journal* by Dr. Whorton, who is a professor of the history of medicine at the University of Washington.[4] He argues that constipation has always been a fearful condition. He notes that the text of an Egyptian papyrus from the sixteenth century BC concerned the poisoning of the body by waste in the colon. Indeed, this autointoxication theory gained more precedence when bacteria were discovered and when it was recognized that the large bowel has lots of bacteria in it. Could these bacteria poison the body? People in the early twentieth century believed so; they feared that constipation could reduce one's life span and linked constipation to many of the unexplained diseases of the day, including what are now recognized to be functional gastrointestinal diseases (including IBS). To combat this fear of colonic intoxication, all sorts of laxative treatments and devices were developed. In the 1920s and '30s, All-Bran cereal was introduced actually to fight this problem. (Another cereal of the time was marketed as DinaMite!) There were electrical stimulators and obscene dilators, massage machines, and colonic irrigations, all developed to combat what some were calling civilization's curse, the constipated bowel. Colonic irrigation survives to this day, of no proven help. We now know that the theory of autointoxication is absolute nonsense, and there is certainly no evidence that being constipated shortens one's life. However, this still hasn't stopped some people, even today, from sometimes going to extreme lengths to fix their bowel regularity if they perceive it is not normal.

We all tend to feel so much better if we can have good regular bowel movements. Indeed, we are often taught that this is important by our parents and have this instilled in us from childhood. The trouble is, bowel normality is pretty variable. Ninety-five percent of the general population will have a bowel movement anywhere from three times a day to three times per week. This frequency is called normal because only 5% of the population is outside this range. If you happen to have either more or fewer bowel movements, even if you experience no other symptoms, you are no longer considered normal, but this does not mean that you have any type of disease. Indeed, if you have absolutely no other symptoms and have always had the same bowel frequency, don't worry; you don't need anything special done. On the other hand, people with IBS often experience quite variable bowel patterns that can come and go and hence be terribly distressing. Indeed, a lack of predictability in regard to one's bowel habits is one of the issues that frequently worry people with this problem. Still, there is no such thing as a normal number of bowel movements per week in reality; what is normal is in the eye of the beholder.

Part of your bowel behavior is under the control of your brain and can be changed. For example, if you suppress the urge to go have a bowel movement and do this repeatedly, you can train yourself to become constipated. An experiment in healthy people confirmed this; medical students were asked to suppress going to the bathroom to pass stool for 4 days, and this did lead to temporary constipation.[5] Moreover, their stomachs also emptied more slowly; hence, you can change your body function with bad habits! Changing the signaling from the bowel to the brain can lead to long-term alterations. However, this can be reversed in some cases with a special form of training called biofeedback (see page 109).

It is very important, therefore, not to delay going to the bathroom when you feel the urge. It is also important to relax and allow sufficient and unhurried time to have a bowel movement. On the other hand, straining excessively or trying to force your bowels to empty more often than they need to will only make things worse and may even damage the muscles and nerves that control bowel function. Taking laxatives just because you want to have a bowel movement every day isn't necessarily a good thing for your body; indeed, it may make your bowel problems temporarily worse. (Laxatives are discussed in Chapter 7.)

EXERCISE: I HATE IT, BUT SHOULD I DO IT?

"I have never taken any exercise except sleeping and resting."
(Mark Twain, 1835–1910)

For the mind and spirit, I believe exercise is essential. Exercise stimulates the immune system (which may be abnormally activated in the bowels of some people with IBS). Exercise reduces stress and can be truly fun and relaxing as well. It can be positive in terms of healing. Exercise is also good for helping you to reduce weight. It may give structure to your day, and it can be a great boredom reliever. While there is no direct evidence that a lack of exercise causes IBS, patients often tell me that adding exercise to their normal routine really helps them manage their symptoms better. This is particularly the case if you also feel low in energy and are having problems with stress aggravating your bowel symptoms. We have observed that people with IBS who exercise have a better quality of life despite their symptoms. We have also found that those who are overweight are more likely to suffer with diarrhea rather than constipation; maybe losing weight through regular exercise helps reduce diarrhea although this is not established.

Almost any type of exercise can be helpful. This includes meditation and yoga as well as stretching, strengthening exercises, and aerobic activity. A key issue is to find something that you like to do, and do it regularly. Try different types of activity if you can, to maintain your interest. Group exercise activities may be the most helpful because they provide a level of support and friendship that can only be beneficial. Consider joining a gym and going often. However, make sure that you don't start exercising vigorously if you have other health problems, such as heart or lung disease, and haven't spoken with your doctor. If you possibly can, make sure you try exercising, and plan to do it for life!

PELVIC MUSCLE EXERCISES

Several different problems can lead to weakness of the pelvic muscles that help control bladder and bowel function. A number of exercises have been developed, particularly for women who have weak pelvic-floor muscles and leak urine when they cough, laugh, or exercise (this is called stress urinary incontinence). The set of exercises commonly called Kegel exercises are done by contracting or squeezing the pelvic-floor muscles to make them stronger and thereby reduce the problem of urine leakage. In addition, strengthening these muscles can sometimes be helpful for people with other pelvic-floor muscle problems such as leakage of stool (which can also occur in those with urine leakage). Stool leakage affects about 1 in 20 people with IBS. These exercises may also sometimes help people who abnormally strain the muscles around the anus when they try to have a bowel movement, which blocks the stool from coming out. Pelvic muscle exercises, combined with other treatments, can help lead to improvement in all aspects of the muscle function down at the bottom end.

To identify the key muscles, imagine you are tightening the muscles around the anus to keep from passing gas. When you squeeze these muscles around the anus and bladder area, try to feel as if you are lifting or drawing in the muscles down there without moving your abdomen or legs. Remember to relax completely after tightening the muscles.

So, lets practice. First, empty your bladder. Then go somewhere quiet where you can concentrate on doing these exercises properly. Sit down or stand or lie, whichever is most comfortable for you. Breath regularly. Tighten the muscles for 5 seconds, and then relax them for 5 seconds; do this ten times. Then tighten the muscles for just 3 seconds, and then relax them for 3 seconds; do this ten times. Repeat the same exercise set three times during the day and again in the evening. You might feel some soreness around the anal area at the beginning, but this usually settles down. You may also find it difficult to contract the muscles for more than a second or two to begin with, but practice will improve their strength, which is the whole idea of the exercise program.

It takes 6 to 12 weeks for improvement to occur, and as with any muscle training program, you must be patient if you want to see success. After this period (assuming you have done the exercises correctly and consistently), there should be some improvement. If there is, then consider doing the exercises at least three times a week to maintain any benefit. Pilates also teaches this exercise and can help if practiced regularly. Try Kegel exercises if you think the muscles down there might be weak; you may be amazed by the results.

BIOFEEDBACK

In a sense, this treatment approach aims to retrain someone who is having difficulty with passing stool because the voluntary muscles around the anus contract when they shouldn't. If you strain a lot, have the feeling of a blockage in the anus to pass stool, feel incompletely emptied, or feel the need to press around the anus, you could have a pelvic muscle problem that is blocking defecation. This can be tested with a simple balloon that is placed in the rectum (during what are called anorectal manometry studies) or with a special radiographic (x-ray) procedure called defecating proctography or by magnetic resonance imaging (MRI).

Fiber doesn't usually help this problem, but biofeedback can. Biofeedback can also help those with leakage of stool into their underwear, assuming there is no major muscle or nerve damage in this area.

There are a number of different techniques used to teach biofeedback.[6] With one method, you lie on your right side, facing the person who will be conducting the retraining program. A balloon is then inserted into the rectum and filled with some air so that it feels as if the rectum were full. Some small surface electrodes are then placed on the skin near the anal opening. With the squeezing or relaxing of the muscles around the anal area, tracings that increase and decrease with muscle activity can then be seen on a television monitor (this is called an electromyogram [EMG] display). You will then be asked to try to push out the balloon from the anus while watching the monitor screen. If the muscle activity increases (rather than decreases, as it should) when you are trying to pass the balloon out, you will be asked to concentrate on that area and to strain without squeezing the anal muscles closed. It may take a number of attempts before you get used to relaxing rather than squeezing there. You will also be taught to make sure that when you are squeezing your abdominal muscles to pass stool, you are also relaxing the muscles around the anal area, as some people do not strain adequately or strain but contract the muscles around the pelvis area when they should not. Each treatment session lasts about half an hour. The length of training programs vary, but our experience is that preferably ten sessions over 1 to 2 weeks are needed to obtain the best results.

The benefits of biofeedback in IBS patients with constipation remain inadequately documented. However, for many people with severe and unexplained constipation, biofeedback can be helpful. About 75% of people do obtain help with this technique if their pelvic muscles are causing constipation, but some will fail to improve. The quality of the therapist conducting the treatment is very important for the best success rate; for this reason, it is worth seeking out an experienced center at which to have this done. Home training is available for biofeedback once initial sessions have been conducted, and this may be as good as having all of the training done at a specialty center.

The real benefit here for constipation is that biofeedback can lead to long-term improvement for some people, without the need for other treatments. I therefore recommend that you discuss this treatment approach with your doctor if you are suffering with mainly constipation and other treatments have failed. You may need to see a specialist to get a further opinion regarding this approach because family practitioners may have limited experience with biofeedback or testing with anorectal manometry.

SUMMING UP

In my experience, diet really can help, but making this happen is in your hands. Remember to eat regular meals, and try to avoid eating large meals in a stressful environment. Sometimes, symptoms will improve naturally if the use of caffeine, alcohol, or tobacco is reduced or eliminated. Remember that if you do have the urge to move your bowels, respond to this if you can instead of suppressing it, but try not to strain excessively, whatever the situation. Your bowels may naturally want to move only a few times per week or less, and this may be quite normal and certainly will not cause you any harm. It is your body, and you can learn to control some of its functions and hence reduce or possibly even eliminate many of the symptoms that you are experiencing.

Take-Home Messages

- Digestion is usually normal in IBS, but diet can help the symptoms.
- Increase your dietary fiber slowly; if you rush, the symptoms may well get worse.
- Try fiber supplements if adding natural fiber in the diet fails; begin slowly!
- Drink plenty of fluids with fiber supplementation.
- Excess gas may respond to a change in diet.
- If you belch all the time, you are swallowing air; recognizing this can help you to stop it.
- Lactose intolerance is common but often is not the cause of IBS-like symptoms. You can find out if it is by consuming no lactose for 2 weeks; if lactose is the cause, your symptoms will go away.
- Exercise improves well-being in people with IBS.
- Biofeedback can be useful for difficult constipation, especially if you have pelvic-floor dysfunction; you will need to go to a gastroenterology center for diagnosis and treatment.

CHAPTER 6

ALTERNATIVE TREATMENTS: WHAT WORKS AND WHAT DOESN'T

"There are some ideas so wrong that only a very intelligent person could believe in them." (George Orwell, 1903–1950)

Complementary and alternative medicine has been defined by the National Institutes of Health in the United States as a group of diverse medical and health care systems, practices, and products that are not presently considered to be part of conventional medicine. Among these approaches are actual alternative medical systems such as homeopathy or ayurvedic medicine; mind-body interventions such as yoga, tai chi, and meditation; so-called biologically based therapies such as herbal treatment or megadose vitamin therapy; manipulative and body-based methods such as chiropractic; and image therapy such as magnetic therapy or reiki.

About one-third of US adults regularly use complementary and alternative medicine, and its use is increasing. Indeed, two-thirds of American adults have used some type of complementary and alternative medicine therapy at some time. However, the majority of people never tell their physician that they are using these therapies, which is a pity because not only do physicians need to be educated, but these therapies sometimes have toxicities; unless the physician knows the patient is on the treatment, any toxicity may not be picked up until it is too late. I have seen cases of liver failure (and death) from the use of herbal medicines by multiple members of one patient's family. Sales of alternative medicine products in the United States are approximately $3 billion (US), and this is increasing annually by about 10%, which is extraordinary. More (over $21 billion [US]) is being spent for various complementary and alternative medicine professional services; half of this is being paid out of pocket by the patient, which almost makes traditional medicine look inexpensive by comparison (which it is not).

A number of unproven approaches to treating irritable bowel syndrome (IBS) are available. Some of these treatments may well provide some additional benefit. You need to carefully consider not only whether the treatment you want to try will work, but also (and even more important) whether it will cause any adverse reactions you really want to avoid. There are lots of charlatans out there who would be happy to take your money to treat you with an unproven therapy. So it really must be "patient beware" when you seek alternative treatments.

HERBAL PRODUCTS AND HERBAL MEDICINE

"No herb ever cures anything, it is only said to cure something. This is always based on the testimony of somebody called Cuthbert who died in 1678. No one ever says what he died of." (Miles Kington, 1983)

A number of different herbal products for people with IBS-type symptoms have been recommended by various practitioners of alternative medicine, but the evidence that most of them work remains extremely limited. Furthermore, many of the preparations labeled as one thing are not particularly well purified, and different manufacturers may produce different strengths, which makes comparisons and studies very difficult in practice. However, there is some evidence, at least for some treatments.

Digestive enzymes include papaya extract, lactase, ox bile extract, and (by prescription) pancreatic enzymes. These are often taken by people with IBS. There are testimonials that some of these types of treatments work but no decent evidence that they are in fact better than placebo. It might be worth trying pancreatic enzymes if you have a lot of diarrhea; if they work, however, you should see a physician to make sure you don't have a problem with the pancreas itself that may be better treated with other methods. At this stage, digestive enzymes are of unproven benefit but remain of some interest.

An *ayurvedic preparation* (containing *Aegle marmelos* Correa plus *Bacopa monnieri* Linn) has been tested in one study. For IBS, this preparation seemed to be better than placebo even though no other studies are available.[1] This work was done in India and has not yet been repeated elsewhere to confirm the results; I am skeptical because of the limited evidence at this time.

Ginger and *aloe* are actually marketed as treatments of IBS in some places, but there is absolutely no controlled-trial evidence that they work for this condition. I doubt it! Similar compounds that small uncontrolled studies have suggested as having some possible benefit for IBS patients include artichoke leaf extract, changjitai, bitter candytuft (*Iberis amara*), and Padma Lax.[2] However, again the lack of evidence is of concern, and the potential toxicity of many of these preparations is unclear. There is really no evidence that vitamins or homeopathy helps people with IBS, and I don't like anyone to take vitamins in large doses, because toxicity is possible.

A more promising treatment for IBS comes from traditional *Chinese herbal medicine.* With Dr. Allan Bensoussan, an expert in Chinese herbal medicine, we conducted a proper double-blind randomized placebo-controlled trial testing different Chinese herbs in patients with IBS in Sydney, Australia.[3] We wanted to be absolutely sure no one knew what they were getting, so we encapsulated the herbs in pills. One group got the placebo herbs, another group got standard doses of the herb combination we chose, and a third group got individualized doses of the herbs, in capsules that looked identical (Figure 6-1). Because the herbs were encapsulated away from the prescribing herbalist, neither the herbalist nor the patients knew which type of pill the patients were actu-

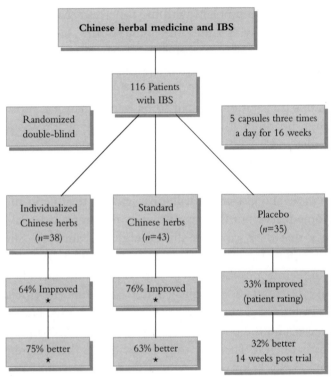

Figure 6-1: Chinese herbal medicine and irritable bowel syndrome (IBS). Asterisk (*) denotes a statistically significant result. Reproduced with permission from Bensoussan et al.[3]

ally getting. The work was published in the prestigious *Journal of the American Medical Association*, and a list of the different herbs included in the formulation appears in Table 6-1. Note that there were 20 different herbs, all of which were considered by the experts to add value in the treatment of the IBS symptom complex. These herbs included all sorts of different substances, including two different seed products.

I was a skeptic (good scientists are taught to be open-minded skeptics early in their career); I believed that such a combination would not work in IBS, but I was wrong.[3]

Patients rated the placebo as working about one-third of the time, which was the expected result. Interestingly, in both the standard and individualized therapies, approximately two-thirds to three-quarters of the patients actually improved, which was a substantially better result than was achieved with placebo. Fourteen weeks after the completion of the study, two-thirds or more of those who received Chinese herbal medicine still felt improved, compared with only one-third of the patients on placebo, and the result was only slightly better in those receiving an individualized formulation rather than a standard formulation. Of course, one pos-

Table 6-1: Chinese Herbal Medicine Standard Formulas (Capsule Ingredients)

Chinese Name	Pharmaceutical Name	Powdered Herb (%)
Dang Shen	*Codonopsis pilosulae*, radix	7.0
Huo Xiang	Agastaches seu pogostemi, herba	4.5
Fang Feng	*Ledebouriellae sesloidis*, radix	3.0
Yi Yi Ren	Coicis lachryma-jobi, semen★	7.0
Chai Hu	*Bupleurum chinense*	4.5
Yin Chen	*Artemesiae capillaris*, herba	13.0
Bai Zhu	*Atactylodis macrocephalae*, rhizoma	9.0
Hou Po	*Magnoliae officinalis*, cortex	4.5
Chen Pi	*Citri reticulatae, pericarpium*	3.0
Pao Jiang	*Zingiberis offinicinalis*, rhizoma	4.5
Qin Pi	Fraxini, cortex	4.5
Fu Ling	*Poriae cocos, sclerotium* (Hoelen)	4.5
Bai Zhi	*Angelicae dahuricae*, radix	2.0
Che Qian Zi	Plantaginis, semen★	4.5
Huang Bai	Phellodendri, cortex	4.5
Zhi Gan Cao	*Glycyrrhizae uralensis*, radix	4.5
Bai Shao	*Paeoniae lactiflorae*, radix	3.0
Mu Xiang	Saussureae seu vladimirae, radix	3.0
Huang Lian	Coptidis, rhizoma	3.0
Wu Wei Zi	Schisandrae, fructus	7.0

Adapted from Bensoussan A et al.[3]
★This means seed in botany.

itive trial does not prove anything. However, this is well recognized as the best trial of Chinese herbal medicine that has been done to date just about anywhere. The challenge remains to identify the key components of this complex herbal formula that may really be benefiting patients. Further work on toxicity is also needed although no serious side effects occurred in this trial.

It is too soon to widely recommend Chinese herbal medicine for IBS, but it is a consideration. If you do seek such care, you should discuss this with a qualified herbalist (which raises the problem of finding one who has the training and expertise to possibly help you safely). I personally do not recommend Chinese herbal medicine for my patients with IBS yet although I will discuss the results of this study with them and consider the option if they wish it strongly. I always emphasize that there may be serious side effects from Chinese herbs (as with any drug). I also tell my patients that any benefits shown in this trial may not apply to them individually.

Licorice comes from a dried plant, and there are different types of licorice, depending on the source (Spanish, Russian, or Persian). Licorice is available in sweets, soft drinks, and chewing tobacco. It is also used in cough mixtures. It does have some antiinflammatory properties as well as having some antispasmodic and laxative affects. Hence, licorice sometimes seems to help people with IBS although there have been no randomized trials with licorice for this condition. Interestingly, licorice did promote healing of peptic ulcer disease although peptic ulcer disease is now treated effectively with antibacterial therapy for *Helicobacter pylori* (see page 10). Licorice can have some side effects if taken in large doses. It can lead to some fluid retention, which can affect people with heart conditions. It can also cause some muscle weakness and headache, as well as lead to missed menstrual periods.

REFLEXOLOGY AND ACUPUNCTURE

A few other alternative medicine methods have been tested for their effect in IBS in proper clinical trials. In a single small trial, reflexology applied to the foot was of no benefit for IBS patients[4]; forget this approach right now.

Acupuncture applied to the colonic meridian (L1 to L4) was shown to be better than sham (fake) acupuncture.[5] In another trial, with 25 patients, no benefit of acupuncture could be demonstrated, but the number of patients studied might have been too small for any benefit to have been detected.[6] We have also looked at the effects of acupuncture on colon function but have been unimpressed.[7] This approach looks rather unpromising at this stage. Still, acupuncture has been shown to be useful for back pain and could therefore perhaps benefit some patients with IBS whose pain is poorly controlled. Proper studies are needed to determine if this is true or not.

IMPROVED SLEEP

There is now evidence that sleep is disturbed in IBS. Sleep studies have been done in the laboratory, measuring the brain's electrical activity as well as the normal sleep phases in IBS, and most of these studies suggest that all of this is normal. However, people with IBS commonly report that they are not obtaining a good night's sleep.[8] It appears that it is the quality of sleep that is abnormal rather than the patterns of sleep.[9]

So what can you do to get a good night's sleep? Some tips that can be helpful are listed below. One thing you should consider avoiding is taking regular sleeping tablets. Unfortunately, although these occasionally can be helpful, you have a problem if you are using them every day; you may be dependent on the pills. Some people who sleep poorly suffer from a specific sleep disorder (such as obstructive sleep apnea, in which the airway becomes blocked off during sleep). However, the majority of people with insomnia do not have a specific sleep disorder but have learned bad habits that can be unlearned.

Help by preparing yourself to sleep well, reserving the hour before bedtime for only quiet activities. It is important to have a bedtime ritual because your body will learn by this ritual that it is indeed time to sleep and will get set up to do so. (The brain's clock is quite accurate; this is why some people don't need an alarm clock to wake up.) If you don't feel sleepy and haven't been able to sleep for a half hour after going to bed, get up and do something quiet; avoid any stimulating activity, and then go back to bed when you feel sleepier.

Keep the bedroom lighting appropriate, and keep the room adequately cool, but be sure it is warm in the bed. Make sure that the clock is out of sight during the night; sometimes, the clock can be distracting. Watching television in bed as well as eating or drinking in bed can be a problem if you are having insomnia, so avoid these habits. Try to keep the bedroom quiet, and use a fan or other sound-producing device if you are troubled by outside noises. Make sure that you have a comfortable bed with clean linen that you like sleeping in.

Keep focusing on pleasant images when you go to bed. Try to find a time to relax, and learn to do progressive muscle relaxation exercises (see page 124) either when you go to bed or in the late evening. Don't drink any caffeine or any other beverages that may stimulate you during the evening before you go to bed. Indeed, decaffeinated coffee can sometimes be stimulating, so try to avoid this too if sleeping is a problem. If you usually need to get up to go to the bathroom during the night to pass urine, try not to drink any liquids after 7:00 pm.

Remember, some people need much less sleep than others required. There are some people who live with only a few hours of sleep although most adults need 7 to 8 hours. If you are able to function well with little sleep, this doesn't mean that there is anything wrong. Indeed, I seriously envy people who can get away with only a few hours of sleep at night and function effectively during the day; it would help me in my job.

If you nap during the day regularly, this may seriously interfere with your ability to sleep at night, so try to avoid napping if you know this is a problem. Stress can make sleeping difficult. Indeed, stress can be one of the major factors causing insomnia. If stress is an issue for you, address it by doing relaxation exercises and seeing your doctor.

Alcohol can also induce poor sleep. It may make you sleepy initially, but then you may wake up very early because of the alcohol's effect on the brain. If this is a problem for you, don't drink alcohol after 7:00 pm.

Try to exercise regularly as this will make your body tired and therefore help you to sleep. Try to get up at the same time every morning, even if you have gone to bed at a slightly different hour than usual, because it is so important to establish daytime as well as nighttime routines (monitored by the brain's central clock and under genetic control).

HUMOR THERAPY

"Happiness is good health and a bad memory." (Ingrid Bergman)

It is funny, but humor seems to be therapeutic. Laughing alters our brain temporarily. When we laugh, we reduce or even temporarily abolish stress. Laughing stimulates the heart, lungs, and muscles. It seems to improve our physical well-being. There is no evidence that laughing improves IBS, but because it increases the release of endorphins in the brain and reduces anxiety, it seems likely that laughing would be helpful. We need proper randomized trials, but how could we blind them, I wonder?

How can one seek out humor? Obviously, this is something each individual needs to cultivate. Going to comedy clubs or movies or (even better) spending lots of time with people who make you laugh are things I believe people with IBS should actively seek to do. Discussions with friends or a counselor can sometimes help you laugh at yourself and make you more receptive to amusing things that have happened in your life. Don't forget to make sure that you add humor to every day of your life.

IMAGERY

You may be able to help your body heal by focusing on positive images, at least according to people who have tried this in serious illnesses. In my view, this is a form of hypnotherapy. Whether imagery has any benefit in IBS is unknown, but it is certainly only likely to help rather than hinder one's getting better. Moreover, this is an active way to participate in the healing process, and so I can see nothing wrong with trying it out and seeing what happens.

Try to imagine that the diet you are following or the medications you are using are going to help your intestine function properly. Imagine the peristaltic waves in your intestines moving in a coordinated way and reducing any trapping of gas in your bowel. Imagine the chemicals in your brain and bowel firing in a way that makes the sensation of pain or discomfort die away. Imagine that you are overriding the circuits in your brain that fire when the bowel is stimulated, so that your symptoms just naturally disappear. Try to see the pictures in your mind, and actively think about them while conscientiously undertaking the relaxation techniques you will learn from this book (see page 124). Try to suppress any negative images while you are doing this, and focus to ensure you are feeling calm and totally empowered. Try to do this every day, and make it part of your ritual before bed or when getting up or whenever it suits you.

JOURNALIZING

If you are having troubling symptoms from the bowel, write down their description, along with how you feel about them, an account of your experiences with them, and the thoughts that you are having. Try to do this on a regular basis. It might help you to write poems or stories or even to paint the images that concern you. You are trying to express yourself through writing so that your feelings, reflections, and thoughts become clear. You may identify physical or emotional needs that you didn't realize were there, and you may be able to find ways of addressing them, which may in turn help your condition. Journalizing can help you remember the questions you have about IBS so you can ask you doctor or other experts for answers. If you are having trouble sleeping, this may help you to calm down and be less fearful and anxious.

Keeping a journal is not for everyone, but for those who feel the need, it can be cathartic to write it all down. It may help you to share these journals with close family or friends. Start today if you think this might be a positive step for you.

ART THERAPY

Like journalizing, art therapy is a means of self expression that can be cathartic for those with IBS. Being creative allows hidden feelings to be expressed, especially with the sharing of creative work. It also helps family and friends to better understand the impact of the illness. Whether it has any therapeutic benefit in IBS is unknown, but it is another natural way to potentially promote healing. The International Foundation for Functional Gastrointestinal Disorders (IFFGD) has an impressive collection of artwork by patients with IBS who have very creatively expressed their feeling, fears, and anger about their illness. All of the paintings in this book come from patients with IBS who have contributed to the IFFGD library of art, and it is a great privilege to be able to present a

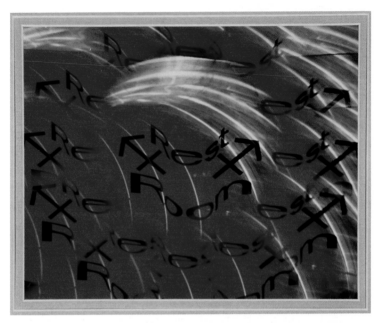

U*R*G*E*N*C*Y, from the the International Foundation for Functional Gastrointestinal Disorders (IFFGD) Art of IBS Collection. Printed with permission from IFFGD (© 2004 IFFGD).

small portion of this work here to illustrate some of the important concepts. Consider trying art therapy for yourself.

PROGRESSIVE MUSCLE RELAXATION

"The nice thing about meditation is that it makes doing nothing quite respectable." (Paul Dean)

Progressive muscle relaxation programs can really help to make you feel calm and quiet. We all have thoughts constantly: try not to think, and it's hard! The mind of a person with IBS is often overactive, perhaps in part because of all of the abnormal signals flooding the brain from the bowel. Relaxation can provide you with a sense of freedom from some of these signals and symptoms and help you learn to cope with the problem. It may take some people time to learn the techniques and to become comfortable with them, but relaxation can be very useful if it is a regular part of your life.

The evidence that relaxation works in IBS is limited, but in controlled trials, relaxation has been shown to lead to symptom improvement (see page 131), suggesting that this is not a technique to casually dismiss. Progressive muscle relaxation is a relaxation technique in which the muscles of the body are relaxed in a set manner, usually starting with the hands and arms and ending with the legs and feet. In progressive muscle relaxation, the body is divided up into a series of large muscle groups, and each group is tensed and then relaxed.

Progressive muscle relaxation can be done by following these simple steps.

First, you will need to learn how to tense and relax the required muscle groups. In progressive muscle relaxation, tension is normally maintained for about 5 seconds, and subsequent relaxation of the muscle group should last 30 seconds. Tense and relax the various muscle groups as follows:

1. Clench the right fist, feeling the tension in the fist and forearm, and then relax… Repeat on the left side.
2. Bend the elbow and tense the biceps, keeping the hands relaxed, and then relax…
3. Straighten the arm and tense the triceps, (the triceps is the muscle on the back of the upper arm) leaving the lower arm supported with the hands relaxed, and then relax…
4. Wrinkle the forehead by raising the eyebrows, and then relax…
5. Bring the eyebrows close together (as in a frown), and then relax…

6. Screw up the muscles around the eyes, and then relax…
7. Tense the jaw by biting (forcing the teeth together), and then relax…
8. With the lips closed, press the tongue hard and flat against the roof of the mouth; notice the tension in the throat, and then relax…
9. Press the lips tightly together (as in a pout), and then relax…
10. Push the head back as far as it will go, and then relax…
11. Press the chin down onto the chest, and then relax…
12. Hunch the shoulders up toward the ears, and then relax…
13. Hunch the shoulders back, and then relax…
14. Pull in the stomach, and then relax…
15. Arch the lower back, and then relax…
16. Tense the buttocks and calves by pressing the feet and toes downward, and then relax…
17. Tense the shins by bending the feet and toes upward, and then relax…

Once you have practiced tensing and relaxing the muscle groups, follow these steps:

1. Find a quiet room and a comfortable chair or bed with good support for the head and shoulders.
2. Close your eyes.
3. Notice your breathing; breathe calmly and regularly first for 2 minutes, and continue this during the relaxation exercises.
4. Go through the tension-and-release exercises listed above twice.
5. At the conclusion, get up slowly, and try to preserve the state of relaxation for as long as possible.

Ideally, progressive muscle relaxation should be practiced once to twice daily, and you will usually need to commit yourself to at least 8 weeks of daily practice to start achieving the long-lasting effects of relaxation.

Tapes or CDs are available to help you do these exercises. Hopefully, these exercises will shift your focus away from the pain or discomfort in your stomach or abdomen, give you the sense that you actually have some control over these symptoms, and refresh you as well as help you heal.

YOGA

Yoga is a very old treatment intervention. It has been practiced for at least 2,000 years. Ancient texts describe yoga as a union of body with mind, mind with spirit, and spirit with consciousness. A comprehensive description of yoga was written by Pantanjali around 200 BC. He described eight integrated steps in the practice of yoga, with physical and breathing exercises constituting two central components.

Yoga exercises should be relaxing. Yoga exercises aim to train and tone different parts of the body, including the abdominal-wall muscles. Indeed, one group of basic yoga exercises are believed to massage and tone not only the abdominal muscles but also the organs inside the abdomen, including the colon. These exercises are done lying down, using different combinations of movement of the legs and abdominal muscles. A key component of these exercises is mental visualization of the muscles and organs that are being exercised or massaged.

In small clinical trials, yoga has been reported to be of benefit to patients with a number of different diseases and conditions, including high blood pressure, asthma, diabetes, osteoarthritis, depression, and stress.[10,11] Unfortunately, there are few studies of yoga in regard to IBS, but on the basis of the limited data, it would seem reasonable to suppose that yoga is useful and is worth trying.[11] Yoga could be helpful because it reduces the symptoms of stress and anxiety and improves the tone of the abdominal muscles. Furthermore, if imagery is used while doing the exercises, it may be possible to further induce relief of the symptoms of IBS, perhaps even slowing or speeding up the bowel (although this is speculative).

Slow regular deep breathing in combination with physical exercises practiced regularly is believed to help regulate bowel function and thus maybe improve symptoms of IBS, but there is little evidence now that this is the case. Further research in this area is ongoing, however. If you decide to practice yoga, don't forget to find a qualified instructor and to let him or her know that you particularly want to focus on the abdominal muscles and organs. I hope this is helpful for you.

MASSAGE

Massage can be a form of relaxation therapy as well as a form of communication. Massage by a partner, for example, will not only reduce some of the muscle tension that may be aggravating one's stomach pain but also may provide greater intimacy and support. Massage can also help you to feel more refreshed, revitalized, and relaxed. If you do not have a partner who can help you with this, a regular massage therapist may provide helpful support. The abdominal-wall muscles can be quite tense in some people with IBS, perhaps secondary to the underlying bowel dysfunction. Even muscles away from the abdomen can be involved, and many people with IBS complain of symptoms of fibromyalgia, as discussed earlier in this book. Massage may help desensitize some of these hypersensitive muscle areas that induce muscle spasm.

PET THERAPY (ANIMAL-ASSISTED THERAPY)

Animal-assisted therapy is believed to provide a form of psychological support. It may distract you from your stomach pain or discomfort (assuming you like pets, of course). The sense of being needed and loved is a natural human need, and if this it missing in your life, consider buying the kind of pet that you can and want to care for. For example, if you need encouragement to do more exercise, buying a dog could be the ideal approach to making it really happen in your life. I have already discussed how useful adding exercise may be for the control of IBS, so don't dismiss this option. Having a pet may also entertain and stimulate you as well as increase your confidence and self-esteem. We all need love and a sense of purpose; think about pet therapy in your life.

SPIRITUALITY

The role of spirituality in healing and health has always been considered to be important. Some of this spirituality may be expressed in attending a church, in journalizing or art therapy, or in meditation or relaxation therapy. Others may find spirituality with friendship, reading, or experiencing the magnificent natural wonders that surround us. Certainly, in terms of managing chronic pain or discomfort and chronic disabling illness, spirituality does seem to have benefits for those with other conditions and therefore presumably also for those with IBS although specific studies of this remain unavailable. Spirituality may also help reduce feelings of anxiety or depression that can affect people with IBS, as previously discussed. This is a very personal search; specific advice cannot be given, but don't discount the importance of healing the mind when trying to heal the body.

MIND-BODY INTERVENTIONS

> "As far as working with your doctor, that's a laugh…Like the one that told me, 'Tell your brain, you're not in pain.' He should have been a poet!"

Telling your brain to dull the pain is feasible; this is a goal of psychological therapy. A number of psychological treatments have been looked at critically in regard to IBS, but the results have been somewhat mixed (Table 6-2). One of the problems with testing these types of treatments in IBS is that it is virtually impossible to blind either the patient or the therapist to the treatment being given. For example, therapists will know if they are hypnotizing a patient, and patients will usually know whether or not they are being hypnotized; there is no fake (sham) treatment that can hide the therapy fully. This means that study results can be misleading because patients or therapists may unconsciously influence the outcomes.

On the basis of a number of randomized controlled trials, hypnotherapy directed to the bowel has been shown consistently to provide a benefit in people with IBS.[12,13] Prof. Peter

Table 6-2:   Types of Mind-Body Treatment for Irritable Bowel Syndrome

Cognitive behavioral therapy
> Consists of a range of techniques designed to alter patients' responses by teaching them to change the way they think and react to certain events. Techniques include education, relaxation training, thinking modification, graded exposure to normally avoided situations, and problem solving.

Psychotherapy
> Interpersonal process designed to bring about a change in a patient's troublesome feelings, thinking, attitudes, or behaviors. Requires a close patient-therapist relationship so that interpersonal difficulties can be addressed.

Hypnotherapy
> Induction of a state of heightened suggestibility and deep relaxation. It can be used to reduce muscle tension and to relax gastrointestinal muscles. Hypnotic techniques include progressive muscle relaxation, eye fixation, and visual imagery.

Relaxation therapy
> Involves a variety of techniques to help a patient control the physical sensations associated with tension. Common techniques include progressive muscle relaxation, breathing retraining, and biofeedback.

Whorwell from England is an expert in this area and has written most about it. Peter has a hypnotic voice, and I am not surprised that he can hypnotize his patients so effectively (he does this to me in lectures). Peter and his team have been able to show that hypnotherapy can alter some normal functions in the bowel, including bowel sensation and contractions; this implies that it works through altering the brain although the mechanisms are unknown. Peter has shown astounding results, training patients through hypnosis to either speed up or slow down their bowel function, depending on whether they have constipation or diarrhea. Hypnosis can also reduce abnormal bowel sensation patterns in those who have a lot of abdominal pain. Patients' acceptance of the technique is reasonably high, and it is extremely safe. Hypnosis has also been shown to work well for people with nonulcer (functional) dyspepsia.[14] The major problem with hypnosis is finding a practitioner who has sufficient expertise and can do bowel-related hypnosis. I have been impressed by these results and feel that for people who have not been helped by other approaches, hypnosis is an excellent alternative worth pursuing. More research in hypnosis is now needed to determine the best technique and to understand how it works. We are working on it!

Other approaches in the area of mind-body intervention revolve around formal psychotherapy. Again, there are studies suggesting that this approach is better than standard care in the treatment of IBS.[13] Cognitive behavior therapy, for example, is a technique that combines relaxation exercises with teaching the patient how to reduce intrusive thoughts that may affect IBS symptoms. However, the benefits of cognitive behavior therapy have been somewhat unclear, with both positive and negative reports of trials in the literature.[15,16]

A meta-analysis has reported an overall benefit of psychological treatments.[17] These approaches all tend to improve well-being but do not get rid of the stomach or bowel symptoms; you may cope better, but these approaches are not a cure for IBS. Unfortunately, finding a good therapist to help with such mind–body treatment is essential but can be challenging as many therapists have not had specific training or experience in managing IBS.

Take-Home Messages

- Few alternative therapies have been subjected to rigorous testing in IBS patients.
- There remains a lack of evidence for most of these approaches (but some may really work).
- Alternative therapy (eg, herbal therapy) can produce severe adverse effects, depending on what herbs are used; "alternative therapy" does not always mean the therapy is safe.
- Relaxation techniques, hypnotherapy, and other mind–body therapies have a place in treating IBS and can really improve feelings of well-being.

OVER-THE-COUNTER MEDICATIONS: EVIDENCE FOR WHAT WORKS AND WHAT DOESN'T

"The desire to take medicine is perhaps the greatest feature which distinguishes man from animals." (Sir William Osler, 1849–1919)

Walk into any pharmacy, and you will see the shelves loaded with medicines for you to try. But the question is, how do you choose between the different medicines? While none of them have been approved by the US Food and Drug Administration (FDA) for IBS, there are compounds for diarrhea, others for constipation, some for gas, others for indigestion, and still more that claim to aid digestion. In this chapter, we will look at what is out there now and the evidence for any benefit in people with IBS. Alternative medicines were already covered in Chapter 6. There are indeed a number of useful medicines that are available over the counter and that may really be helpful for the short-term control of IBS symptoms, particularly during periods of exacerbation.

FIBER PRODUCTS (BULKING AGENTS)

Fiber was discussed in detail in Chapter 5. There is no doubt that fiber products available over the counter all can aid constipation in people with IBS. They may also firm up the stools if looseness, rather than constipation, is a problem. There seems little to choose among the commercial fiber compounds that are available (Table 7-1). However, a meta-analysis of randomized controlled trials testing fiber products in IBS patients have given us some new guidance. In particular, based on the evidence, fiber products that contain soluble fiber may be most useful. Soluble fiber products include psyllium, ispaghula, and calcium polycarbophil. Psyllium is a very common fiber product (see page 93).

Table 7-1: Examples of Commonly Used Commercially Available Fiber Products

Product	Form	Fiber Content
Metamucil		
Psyllium	Powder	3.4 g/dose*
Psyllium	Wafers	3.4 g/wafer
FiberCon		
Polycarbophil	Tablets	0.5 g/tablet
Fiberall		
Polycarbophil	Tablets	1.0 g/tablet
Psyllium	Wafers	3.4 g/wafer
Psyllium	Powder	3.4 g/tsp
Citrucel		
Methylcellulose	Powder	2.0 g/tbsp

*Regular and sugar-free, 1 tsp; orange and strawberry flavor, 1 tbsp.
Adapted from Zighelboim J, Talley NJ. Irritable bowel syndrome. Gastroenterology 1993;104:1196–201.

Ispaghula is the husk of psyllium and is coarser than other products.

The published meta-analyses on the role of fiber supplements in IBS treatment are of importance. Overall, it appears that fiber is better than placebo in terms of improving constipation in IBS. On the other hand, the abdominal pain or discomfort that people with IBS have may often not improve more with fiber supplements than with placebo, although here the information is mixed and some studies do show a little benefit. The results also showed that soluble fiber supplements (mainly psyllium) were of the greatest benefit whereas insoluble fiber (corn or wheat bran) did not help. Hence, if you are choosing a fiber product, it seems sensible to follow the evidence.

I no longer routinely recommend corn or wheat bran for my patients with IBS, but I do suggest that it is always worth trying one of the soluble fiber supplements, particularly psyllium, which is available in many commercial products in the United States. I do not recommend wheat or corn bran for all my patients because these appear to be more likely to cause gas and bloating and not likely to make other symptoms better.

The benefit of fiber supplements is modest at best, but because of their safety, they are still the first line of treatment. It is very important to start off with a soluble fiber supplement such as psyllium and begin at a low dose, increasing the amount you take very slowly to reduce any bloating or gas problems from the medication. Unfortunately, fiber can increase bloating and gas even if started in a low dose, but it can be worthwhile persisting with the fiber supplement for at least 4 to 8 weeks before giving up (the bloating often settles by then). If fiber products help, then it is reasonable to continue them for life. Many patients take the products for only a short time and cease taking them when the benefit occurs, only to find that the symptoms come back. In my clinical experience, the reinstitution of fiber in this situation doesn't always work as well although why this is the case is unclear.

Psyllium can also have side effects although they are relatively rare. Psyllium can cause potentially severe allergic reactions, including asthma and collapse, but this is very rare. Psyllium can also (rarely) cause a blockage in the esophagus or intestine. Whether psyllium should be used in pregnancy is unclear; as with all medications, it should be stopped during pregnancy unless you are advised otherwise by your doctor.

LAXATIVES

"You have a cough? Go home tonight, eat a whole box of Ex-Lax—tomorrow you'll be afraid to cough." (Pearl Williams)

There are lots of different laxatives, and this is very confusing for people with IBS whose major problem is constipation. Let's discuss the different classes of laxatives (both over-the-counter and prescription products) so we can understand what may or may not help.[1]

Mineral Oil

Mineral oil helps lubricate the stool so that it is softer. However, mineral oil alone generally fails to improve bowel function in people with IBS and, while generally safe, is not something to take routinely. There are no clinical trials of this drug class in IBS. The biggest problem with mineral oil is that people complain of seepage of small amounts of liquid stool into their underpants. The drug can also cause pneumonia occasionally, as well as block the absorption of some of the important fat-soluble vitamins such as vitamin D (needed for healthy bones) and vitamin A (needed for vision).

Stool Softeners

Stool (or fecal) softeners are thought to help reduce hard stools by decreasing the surface tension and increasing the amount of fluid in the stool itself. One of the commonest brands is Colace (dioctyl sodium sulfosuccinate); this compound is also used in ear drops for softening ear wax. Another brand is Surfak (dioctyl calcium sulfosuccinate). In addition to diarrhea, stool softeners can cause abdominal cramping, nausea, and skin rash. Stool softeners usually do little to help the constipation of IBS! This may be because stools may feel hard but are not actually firmer in IBS than in health.

Stimulant Laxatives

Stimulant laxatives work by directly stimulating the nerve endings in the colon, thereby increasing contractions in the bowel as well as stimulating fluid release. For example, castor oil was once widely used by mothers to "regulate" their children's bowels (what a disaster!). There are many different stimulant laxatives on the market, including drug preparations that contain bisacodyl (eg, Fleet laxative, Dulcolax, and Correctol) or senna (eg, Senokot, Perdiem Overnight Relief, Ex-Lax, and Fletcher's Castoria). Also available are combination laxatives such as Senokot-S and Peri-Colace (containing senna and docusate sodium). All of these stimulant laxatives can induce cramping, which is a problem. Senna products can cause asthma and other allergic reactions occasionally. Hepatitis has been reported with heavy use of senna products.

Phenolphthalein is no longer available as an over-the-counter laxative in the United States because of a concern (based on animal experiments) that this particular laxative might damage the bowel in the long term. It has never been fully established that this is the case, but the so-called laxative bowel syndrome (in which the large bowel just no longer works at all because of excessive laxative use) has been extremely rare since the banning of these laxative compounds in the United States. Phenolphthalein also caused cancers in rats and mice, another reason for the withdrawal of this particular drug. However, if you are traveling overseas, there are still some countries where you can get phenolphthalein-containing laxatives, so look carefully at the label before you take anything like this over the long term.

The anthraquinones in laxatives can actually make the colon look blackish, which can be seen with a colonoscopy. This is not otherwise thought to be a problem.

There are no randomized placebo-controlled trials of stimulant laxatives in IBS. The evidence for any benefit is poor for constipation as well.[1] Stimulant laxatives seem to control constipation poorly in IBS, often wear off, and aggravate abdominal discomfort or pain. I don't recommend them routinely, and if used they should not be taken daily.

Osmotic Laxatives

Osmotic laxatives work by drawing fluid from the lining of the bowel so that there is an increase in the water volume in the bowel (the water being then propelled out). Examples include laxatives that contain magnesium citrate or magnesium hydroxide (magnesium-containing drugs cause diarrhea; while aluminum–containing compounds are constipating). It is important to avoid magnesium-containing laxatives such as milk of magnesia if you have any history of major kidney disease or renal failure. This is because magnesium is a heavy metal that can accumulate in the body if the kidneys fail to work properly. Retention of magnesium salts can lead to nausea, vomiting, flushing of the skin, excessive thirst, low blood pressure, drowsiness, confusion, slurred speech, double vision, weakness in the muscles, slow heart rate, and even (rarely) death. Elderly people are more at risk for toxic reactions. Magnesium crosses the placenta, so it must be avoided in pregnancy unless given under strict medical supervision.

Laxatives that contain sorbitol or lactulose are also osmotic laxatives. Sorbitol is a sugar alcohol present in many fruits and vegetables and is prepared commercially in order to lower the amount of glucose needed for sweetening. It can worsen feelings of gas and induce diarrhea, an effect used when it is given as a relatively inexpensive laxative. Lactulose is similar but usually more expensive. Trade names include Duphalac, Chronulac, and Kristalose. Lactulose also works as an osmotic laxative. The taste is somewhat unpleasant to many. Occasionally, lactulose can induce nausea and vomiting but usually only in high doses.

Polyethylene glycol (PEG) is a potent osmotic laxative that has worked well in people with severe constipation in clinical trials although again, no studies have been done in regard to IBS. It is now available over the counter. One brand on the market is MiraLax. Most trials have been short, but there is one study that tested the drug over a 20-week period.[2] PEG certainly increases bowel movements in patients with difficult-to-treat constipation. It is FDA approved for short term use in constipation (2 weeks); I prescribe it for tough cases "off label." Discuss this alternative with your doctor.

How to Choose the Right Laxative

Laxatives have only modest benefits, and any help may wear off over time with some compounds. They are not addictive, but any benefit in IBS is usually small.

You can see that there are a lot of different laxatives; the problem with this group of agents is the lack of evidence that they really work in IBS. However, they can be of help for constipation, and many people do try them. It is generally recommended that one starts with an osmotic laxative; if this fails, then one can try a stimulant laxative. These drugs generally appear to be safe if not used all the time, but you need to discuss the type of laxative you want to use with your physician before embarking on the life-long use of this or any other type of treatment.

ENEMAS AND SUPPOSITORIES

Many patients (particularly men, it seems) do not like the idea of inserting anything into the anus to help with defecation. However, if there is a particular problem with excessive straining and feelings of a blockage in this area, enemas or suppositories can sometimes be beneficial for short-term relief. There are often better alternatives, however. For example, if there is a problem with the muscles around the anal area, blocking defecation, those muscles can be retrained with biofeedback; this is an important idea to consider with one's doctor (see page 109).

ANTIDIARRHEAL DRUGS

A number of over-the-counter drugs are sold to relieve diarrhea, and there is good evidence of what truly works here.

Loperamide

Loperamide (sold as Imodium A-D and Imodium Advanced) is an opiate compound. It does not cross into the brain, so it has none of the euphoric effects seen with opiates used on the street. It is not addictive. Imodium reduces the speed at which material moves through the intestine and also reduces water and electrolyte movement in the bowel; in a sense, it plugs you up temporarily. Its main problem is that it tends to cause constipation, and this can be a real issue with IBS because constipation can be as troubling as diarrhea. Well-done randomized placebo-controlled trials have tested this agent in regard to IBS. They have reported good results in terms of diarrhea but have also shown that the abdominal pain and bloating do not get better on the drug. Side effects of loperamide include, very rarely, acute bowel inflammation. Rarely, an allergic reaction to loperamide can occur, but loperamide is generally a very safe drug.

So how should you use it? It is important to realize that the instructions on the use of this drug from the pharmacy actually don't work terribly well for IBS diarrhea. You should *not* just take the medication after the diarrhea has commenced. It is much better (particularly if the diarrhea is reasonably pre-dictable) to use it as a preventative measure. For instance, if your diarrhea usually happens after breakfast or after a meal or happens when you are likely to become particularly stressed, then take a dose of loperamide before the meal or event. This can be really helpful! Alternatively, I often tell patients to try taking loperamide (one or two 2 mg tablets) first thing in the morning to prevent the morning rush of diarrhea and then at night before going to bed if they are being disturbed during the night with diarrhea. It takes a bit of trial and error to learn how best to use loperamide. Some people need quite high doses of the drug for it to work well for them; here, guidance by a doctor is critical. Loperamide is a very good drug for diarrhea in IBS, and if you have this problem, consider trying it. If you also suffer with some leakage of stool into your underpants, this drug can help because it tightens up the anal muscles.

Lomotil

Another drug that is often tried for diarrhea in IBS is Lomotil, which is actually a combination of two different drugs, namely, diphenoxylate and atropine. The atropine is put in to prevent people from getting too much of the diphenoxylate, which can cause a "high" (if you take too much you get side effects from the atrophine). Only available on prescription, the US Food and Drug Administration indication for this drug is diarrhea, not IBS. There are actually no studies of this drug's use for IBS although it does seem to help some people. It can cause side effects that include dizziness and drowsiness as well as feelings of tiredness. Nausea and vomiting and abdominal pain can also occur. There have been rare reports of serious allergic reactions with the drug, including dilation of the colon and inflammation of the pancreas. It is a useful alternative to loperamide in IBS with diarrhea.

Bismuth Subsalicylate

Although there is a lack of good evidence, another drug that could be useful in IBS treatment is bismuth subsalicylate (eg, Pepto-Bismol). This drug is often used for the prevention of traveler's diarrhea as well as the treatment of nonspecific diarrhea and indigestion. Some people who take this drug for IBS and diarrhea note major improvement. The antibacterial and antiinflammatory properties of bismuth subsalicylate may indeed theoretically reduce the inflammation that can occur in IBS although this is unproven. The main problem with bismuth is that it is a heavy metal; thus, it can potentially cause brain damage if used in high doses in the long term. Outbreaks of encephalopathy (a brain disease), particularly in

France, have been seen with heavy usage of bismuth in the past, so if the drug is taken, it certainly must be taken only for a short period. However, if your type of IBS is one in which you have symptoms only for a few weeks and are then free of symptoms for long periods, a trial of Pepto-Bismol might be worthwhile. If you plan to take it for any prolonged length of time (over 2 days), definitely consult your doctor.

Other Antidiarrheal Drugs

There is no evidence that any other over-the-counter antidiarrheal medications (such as Kaopectate) are of any benefit in regard to IBS.

GAS-REDUCING DRUGS

Gas is a major challenge in the management of IBS, and good agents for helping people with this particular problem are lacking. A number of over-the-counter antigas products are available, but their usefulness is probably not great.

Simethicone

Simethicone is essentially an antibubbling agent and is therefore marketed as a drug for excessive gas. It is usually available in a chewable tablet with an antacid, but one can also buy simethicone capsules. Some of the products that contain simethicone are Gas-X, Mylanta Gas, and Phazyme. Try taking 125 mg during meals. Simethicone can cause diarrhea as well as nausea and vomiting and headaches; a rash is rare. While this is worth a try for the relief of gas in IBS, my patients tell me it usually works poorly for them.

Activated Charcoal

Activated charcoal (eg, CharcoCaps, Charcoal Plus) is used as an antigas agent, but the evidence for its benefit in IBS is even less than that for simethicone. The dose is 1 to 2 tablets taken one-half hour after meals. Charcoal can occasionally cause a blockage in the bowel, which is serious; diarrhea, vomiting, and dark stool will occur with its use in some cases. I don't generally recommend it to help with antigas problems.

PEPPERMINT OIL

A number of essential oils have properties that potentially reduce spasm in the bowel and possibly calm disturbed bowel function. Peppermint oil is obtained by steam distillation of the flower *Mentha x piperita*. The active ingredient in peppermint oil is menthol, which blocks calcium going into the cells. A number of calcium antagonists have been tried in IBS treatment, with mixed results.

A review of the literature and a meta-analysis evaluated eight trials that tested peppermint oil for IBS treatment.[3] Overall, there did appear to be a greater benefit with peppermint oil than with placebo. However, the quality of the studies was judged to be relatively low; thus, the benefit is not absolutely clear-cut, unfortunately. The results led the authors of this meta-analysis to suggest that further well-designed and carefully executed studies were needed to confirm the initial results. This is the conundrum of science; clinical trial evidence cannot prove a premise, but it can disprove it. A large well-done randomized trial whose results were negative would be strong evidence in favor of peppermint oil's not working whereas a large well-designed study whose results were positive would be evidence in favor of the value of peppermint oil but would not prove that it works. We cannot adequately judge the benefit just on the basis of small low-quality randomized controlled trials, even if the data are combined in a meta-analysis.

Peppermint oil is worth a try for the abdominal pain and cramps of IBS. The usual dosage is 0.2 mL three times a day, taken one-half hour to one hour before meals and swallowed whole (not chewed). Peppermint oil should not be taken with alcohol as this can increase its side effects. A number of uncommon reactions with peppermint oil use have been reported, including red skin rashes, headaches, a slow heart rate, muscle spasms, and a feeling of severe unsteadiness; increased heartburn has also been reported. Peppermint oil may worsen asthma. An irregular heartbeat due to atrial fibrillation has also been reported to occur with peppermint ingestion. It is not, therefore, a treatment without risk. Do not take it long term without medical advice.

Hot peppermint teas are an alternative worth trying. Indeed, hot fluids alone may help calm excessive esophageal muscle contractions that cause chest pain and trouble swallowing.[4]

ANTACIDS AND ACID-REDUCING DRUGS

Many antacids are available and may sometimes help with gas and indigestion in IBS. Magnesium-containing antacids cause diarrhea, so if you have mainly constipation, try these antacids. Aluminum-containing antacids, on the other hand, are constipating, so try this type if your problem is diarrhea. Remember, most antacids mix magnesium and aluminum to prevent both diarrhea and constipation! Short-term use of antacids is generally safe, but regular and heavy use should be undertaken under guidance from your doctor.

Two classes of acid-reducing drugs are available over the counter: histamine receptor antagonist drugs and proton pump inhibitors. There are many different histamine receptor antagonists, including ranitidine (Zantac) and cimetidine (Tagamet). These drugs reduce acid secretion and can help some of the indigestion symptoms associated with IBS, particularly heartburn. They work fairly promptly and are most useful if the heartburn or indigestion is an intermittent problem. The doses sold over the counter are relatively low compared to the prescription doses, so if this type of drug is helpful, it is sometimes worthwhile getting a prescription (discuss this with your doctor). Some people who take acid-suppressing drugs report that their bowel symptoms also improve, but whether this is just a placebo response is unknown; there are no proper trials of these agents in IBS treatment.

Side effects with the histamine receptor antagonists are infrequent, but diarrhea, dizziness, tiredness, headache, and rashes can occur. Very rare adverse events include liver damage, blood disorders, inflammation in the pancreas, heart disorders, and the development of a small amount of breast tissue in men. Long-term follow-up of patients taking drugs of this class have shown that they are remarkably safe and can generally be used with real confidence.

A much more potent acid-suppressing drug is the proton pump inhibitor omeprazole (Prilosec), which is now available over the counter in the United States (the over-the-counter dose is the same as the prescription dose, namely, 20 mg). Omeprazole blocks the gastric acid pump that leads to the release of acid into the stomach. Proton pump inhibitors are excellent for controlling heartburn although not everyone will respond adequately. For maximum effect, omeprazole should be taken on an empty stomach 30 minutes before a meal once daily because it works by turning off the stomach's acid pump, which is stimulated by a meal.

Some people with IBS in clinical practice report that their bowel symptoms improve with the use of omeprazole although whether this is a placebo response is unknown. The drug is generally very safe. A few people get abdominal pain with omeprazole, which is obviously a disadvantage. Headaches can occur as well as (rarely) serious skin rashes or an abnormal blood count. A number of other acid-pump blockers are available by prescription.

SIDE EFFECTS VERSUS ALLERGIES

Just because a product is sold over the counter does not mean that it cannot have side effects and even (rarely) serious side effects. Any drug can cause a reaction; this does not necessarily mean there is an allergy to the drug. Many side effects occur because of the pharmacologic action of the compound. For example, a drug that stimulates the bowel to move material through it more quickly (ie, a stimulant laxative) will obviously cause diarrhea in some people, as well as excessive cramps (from the increased abdominal contractions) and nausea, which often accompanies cramping of the abdomen from any cause. It would be wrong to then conclude that because one experiences such side effects, one is allergic to the stimulant laxative; the side effects here are to be expected. If side effects occur, reducing the dose or changing to a different drug in the same drug class can sometimes help. Of course, any drug can also cause rare allergic reactions, and if this happens, one should never be exposed to the compound again. Rashes, breathing problems, collapse, or swelling of the body may be evidence of a true drug allergy.

Take-Home Messages

- Fiber products help constipation and possibly other IBS symptoms but may make gas and bloating worse.
- You need to give a fiber supplement a chance; for some people, it takes weeks to months for a benefit to occur.
- When increasing dietary fiber with fiber supplements, only do so very slowly and steadily.
- Laxatives can help constipation but probably have no benefit for other IBS symptoms; osmotic laxatives are safe and can be used if fiber fails.
- Antidiarrheal drugs such as Imodium help relieve diarrhea but not pain or bloating from IBS.
- Peppermint oil may help cramping in the abdomen.

DRUG TREATMENTS: EVIDENCE FOR WHAT WORKS

*"I do not think that my GI [gastrointestinal] doctor under-
stands the severity of my condition, though I am happier with
him than I have been with any others I have seen. He is the
only one who has provided any solution that helped. He has
referred to my condition as 'uncomfortable' and 'annoying';
understatements, to say the least."*

We have already discussed the placebo response in regard to
irritable bowel syndrome (IBS). The results of clinical trials
that have been done with people with this condition indicate that at least 3 in 10 people with IBS who are given a
dummy treatment (ie, placebo) will gain some benefit.[1]
Let's then review the evidence from the medical literature
that drugs that are currently widely prescribed by physicians for IBS actually work. You may be surprised by some
of the answers you will find here; for many of the treatments doctors prescribe, there is either limited or no evidence that they work. On the other hand, there is much
stronger evidence in favor of newer drugs that have been
released for IBS treatment. You will also be interested to
know that most drugs have side effects that can be worri-
some. For most people, the side effects are mild if they
occur at all, but unfortunately, any drug with pharmacologic actions in the body will also affect other systems in the
body, occasionally leading to serious problems, even (rarely)
death. This is where doctors and patients need to weigh the
potential benefits of a treatment against the risks. If the
drug has no benefit and yet there is a potentially serious
risk, then one really should not use it. On the other hand,
if the drug is particularly effective but serious side effects
can still occur occasionally, the decision to use the medication can be much more difficult. This is always a personal

decision, and it is very important to discuss the issue carefully with your physician, who can help guide you through the problem. It is certainly sometimes worth taking the risk that a medication will have serious side effects if it will improve your quality of life substantially.

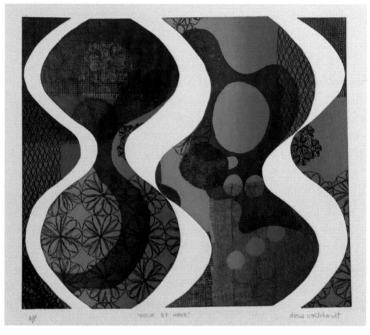

Hour by Hour, from the International Foundation for Functional Gastronintestinal Disorders (IFFGD) Art of IBS Collection. Printed with permission from the IFFGD (© 2004 IFFGD).

TYPES OF DRUGS USED FOR IRRITABLE BOWEL SYNDROME

Antispasmodics

Many doctors prescribe medicines that they hope can reduce the spasms of the bowel that are thought to occur in some people with IBS. Even though bowel spasm is no longer believed to play a major role in the symptoms, prescription of these drugs continues. In the United States, the available drugs are all of one type (anticholinergics); the trade names used for some of these compounds are listed in Table 8-1. However, the evidence that these drugs are actually better than placebo is remarkably limited as there have been only a very few trials.[1] Of the three available studies, two showed no significant benefit of the drug over placebo whereas one of the studies showed that IBS symptoms did improve when compared with the placebo (but used a high dose leading to very frequent adverse reactions).

In Europe and other parts of the world, other antispasmodic agents are available. A meta-analysis of all these drugs suggested that overall, antispasmodics do provide a small amount of benefit (compared with placebo) in improving both the overall symptoms and abdominal pain of IBS.[2] The most useful drugs include mebeverine and trimebutine, but neither of these drugs is currently available in the United States. You

Table 8-1: Some Antispasmodics for Treatment of Irritable Bowel Syndrome

Generic Name	Trade Name	Form	Dose (adult)
Hyoscyamine	Levsin	Tablets, elixir, drops	0.125–0.25 mg★
Hyoscyamine	Levsinex	Timed-release capsules	0.375–0.75 mg twice daily
Tincture of belladonna		Drops	0.2–0.75 mL★†
Dicyclomine	Bentyl	Tablets, capsules, syrup	20–40 mg★
Propantheline	Pro-Banthine	Tablets	7.5 mg–15 mg★

★Before meals and at bedtime.
†0.1 mL = 2 drops.
Adapted from Zighelboim J, Talley NJ. Irritable bowel syndrome. Gastroenterology 1993; 104:1196–201.

might ask why these drugs are not available in the United States, and the answer is, partly because of marketing forces. When drug patents expire, it usually is no longer economically viable for drug companies to bring those drugs to market, and this is the problem with these older drugs for IBS. It seems a shame to have relatively safe drugs that appear to provide at least some benefit in IBS available for people elsewhere but not in the United States. Only political action could change this situation although the lobbying forces that would be brought to bear from big pharma trying to protect its substantial profit margins against such action would likely be considerable.

Antidiarrheal Drugs

Antidiarrheal drugs are effective agents for diarrhea in IBS, but they are often used incorrectly (see Chapter 7). The drug that has actually been tested in IBS is loperamide, most commonly known by the trade name Imodium. Loperamide is an excellent and safe drug.[2] It actually increases the absorption of water and electrolytes in the bowel; as well, it reduces the secretion of fluid into the bowel and slows the time it takes fluid to move through the bowel. All of these effects are of benefit in diarrhea. In addition, loperamide also can help contract the anal muscle area, so this drug can be excellent for the problem of severe urgency (being unable to reach the bathroom in time). All of the randomized trials of this drug in IBS have indicated that it helps diarrhea. Unfortunately, it does not relieve abdominal pain or other IBS symptoms. It is very important that this drug be taken in the correct fashion when used for IBS symptoms. The best way to take it is to use it to prevent attacks of diarrhea. For many people with IBS who get diarrhea after breakfast, it is worth taking the medication as soon as one wakes up in the morning. Another dose before lunch or before supper can be very helpful. Taking the drug after diarrhea occurs (which is recommended on the packaging) can be quite unhelpful.

Another prescription medication that is helpful is diphenoxylate (Lomotil). However, there are no controlled trials of its use in IBS treatment although certainly it is helpful in practice, particularly if loperamide doesn't work. A drug to avoid is codeine phosphate (available only by prescription). The problem with codeine is that although it works, it can lead to dependence and therefore cannot be recommended.

There is some evidence that a small number of people with IBS actually have the problem of being unable to absorb all the bile salts that come from the liver and flow into the small bowel. When this occurs, the bile salts wash over into the colon and actually cause fluid to squirt out of the cells, causing diarrhea. The use of an agent that mops up these bile salts, such as cholestyramine (e.g. Questran Lite) can help reduce the diarrhea although no controlled trials in IBS exist. Cholestyramine is used to reduce cholesterol, but it can help diarrhea for some people with troublesome IBS and diarrhea who have not responded well to the other agents discussed above.

Antidepressants

Many patients become very frightened or upset when their physician suggests they should try an antidepressant medication for their IBS symptoms, but you should not feel this way. Antidepressants, of course, are used for depression. While the US Food and Drug Administration has not approved antidepressants for IBS, these drugs do appear to be useful for IBS treatment, but not because they work for depression. Indeed, antidepressants do work in the brain and in the bowel; they seem to actually help reduce pain signals coming from the bowel and can therefore be of benefit, particularly for abdominal pain.[2,3] Table 8-2 lists some antidepressants that may be prescribed for treatment of IBS.

There are a number of different classes of antidepressants. The tricyclic antidepressants are older agents, but they can

Table 8-2: Some Antidepressants That May Be Prescribed for Treatment of Irritable Bowel Syndrome (Adults)

Generic Name	Trade Name	Usual Daily Dose (mg)
Amitriptyline	Elavil	25–75
Desipramine	Norpramin	25–75
Doxepin	Sinequan	25–75
Imipramine	Tofranil	25–75
Nortriptyline	Aventyl, Pamelor	25–75
Trazodone	Desyrel	100–150 (in divided doses)
Fluoxetine	Prozac	20–40 (once daily)
Citalopram	Celexa	20 (once daily)
Escitalopram	Lexapro	10 (once daily)

Adapted from Zighelboim J, Talley NJ. Irritable bowel syndrome. Gastroenterology 1993; 104:1196–201.

benefit IBS. For example, a treatment trial with the tricyclic antidepressant desipramine (Norpramin) showed that 60% of people on this agent obtained a benefit, compared with 47% of those on placebo.[2] The dose that is used for IBS is typically much lower than the dose that is usually used for depression, presumably because the agent works in a different way for IBS. These drugs take time to work; at least 1 month on treatment should pass before the drug is considered a failure and stopped. Taking the medication for only a few days is just not adequate as it takes time for the agent to affect the body's chemicals. The problem with the tricyclic antidepressants is that they can cause side effects, sometimes serious. These include constipation, nausea, weight change (up or down), fatigue, heart problems, liver toxicity, blood count changes, and other rare events.

Many physicians (including I)will use this type of drug in someone with moderate or severe IBS for whom other treatments have failed; this is because the benefits tend to outweigh the risks of therapy in such a case. Many of my patients (although not all) who have taken antidepressants for IBS have done very well. Taking an antidepressant needs to be discussed carefully with your doctor but is worth considering, particularly if your symptoms are affecting your quality of life severely.

Some of the newer antidepressants are of uncertain benefit in IBS, but they are often used because they have fewer side effects.[2] The agents that have been most often tried are the selective serotonin reuptake inhibitors such as fluoxetine (Prozac). However, the evidence that this class of agents really works in IBS treatment is very limited and conflicting. There are other classes of antidepressants that have not been tested for IBS but could be useful. Again, a physician with expertise in the use of this class of agents can be very helpful for people with very troublesome IBS. It seems that the individual response to different agents varies enormously (probably partly for genetic reasons), so there is an element of trial and error in determining the best one to use. It is important to recognize that the use of antidepressants does not lead to any addiction or dependence.

A number of herbs (such as St. John's wort) have been tested as treatment for depression[4]; however, there are as yet no studies of their use for IBS.

Anxiety-Reducing Medications

Some people want to reduce the anxiety that is associated with their IBS and try agents that actually work as antianxiety medications. These can be useful for very short-term treatment of the anxiety, but they probably don't help other IBS symptoms. They can have significant side effects (such as causing one to sleep poorly) as well as lead to dependency and are therefore not recommended.

Kava, derived from a plant and used in a traditional drink in the South Pacific islands, can help anxiety in the short term,[4] but again there are no studies of its use for IBS.

Tegaserod

Tegaserod (Zelnorm in the USA or Zelmac in other parts of the world) is a newer agent that was released for the treatment of IBS with constipation in women. It has also been approved by the US Food and Drug Administration for women and men with chronic constipation under age 65. It acts on the serotonin type 4 receptor, stimulating it (Figure 8-1). This stimulation increases contractions in the bowel propelling the contents forward (Figure 8-2), stimulates fluid secretion, and

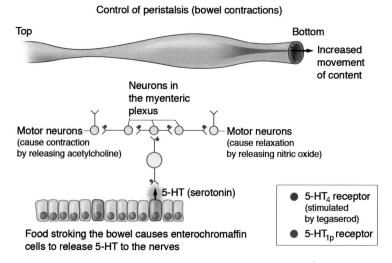

Figure 8-1: Tegaserod stimulates bowel peristalsis by stimulating serotonin receptor type 4 (5-HT4). Note the intricate circuits in the nerves that control the bowel. Adapted with permission from American Gastroenterological Association, Grider JR, et al. 5-Hydroxytryptamine 4 receptor agonists initiate the peristaltic reflex in human, rat, and guinea pig intestine. *Gastroenterology* 1998;115:370-80. Adapted from © MedReviews, LLC with permission of MedReviews, LLC. Gershon MD. "Serotonin and its implication for the management of irritable bowel syndrome" *Reviews in Gastroenterology Disorders* 2003; 3 (Suppl 2): S25-34. *Reviews in Gastroenterological Disorders* is a copyrighted publication of MedReviews, LLC. All rights reserved.

Tegaserod in IBS speeds up colon transit

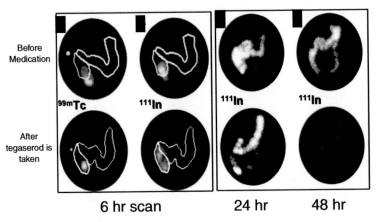

Figure 8-2: A nuclear medicine test of colon transit shows that the colon moves material in it faster after treatment with tegaserod. (IBS = irritable bowel syndrome; [111]In = indium 111; Rx = medication; [99m]Tc = technetium 99m) Reproduced with permission from Prather CM, Camilleri M, Zinsmeister AR, et al. Tegaserod accelerates orocecal transit in patients with constipation-predominant irritable bowel syndrome. Gastroenterology 2000;118:463-8.

blocks pain signals moving from the bowel to the brain. Clinical trials have shown that this drug is clearly better than placebo for IBS and constipation; about two–thirds of users have improvement, but the placebo response is also quite high (Figure 8-3).[1,2,5]

The drug appears to be relatively safe; diarrhea and headache are the major side effects reported. Rare reports of bleeding from the bowel in patients taking this drug (due to low blood supply to the bowel, causing damage) have appeared in the medical literature although cause and effect has not been proven; if you start to see blood in your stools, you should see your physician promptly. Any drug can have very serious side effects rarely, and with new drugs, these may

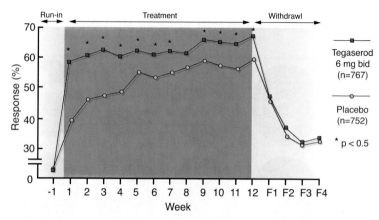

Figure 8-3: Results of a randomized double-blind placebo-controlled trial of tegaserod versus placebo in women with constipation and irritable bowel syndrome (IBS). Tegaserod beat placebo in this study. (bid = twice daily) Reproduced with permission from Novick, J, Miner P, Krause R, et al. A randomized, double-blind, placebo-controlled trial of tegaserod in female patients suffering from irritable bowel syndrome with constipation. Aliment Pharmacol Ther 2002;16:1877–88.

not yet be appreciated for a long time, so keep this in mind. Always discuss safety issues with your doctor, and read the package insert carefully.

The usual dosage of tegaserod is 6 mg twice a day. However, the drug does not work for people who have diarrhea, and its benefit for people who alternate between diarrhea and constipation is unclear. Furthermore, the benefit of the drug in men is unknown. Physicians sometimes prescribe it for men, anyway (this is called "off-label" prescribing); some seem to benefit. Tegaserod is a useful medication for people for whom fiber and bulking agents have failed, but it doesn't work for everyone.

Alosetron

In the United States, alosetron (Lotronex) is approved by the US Food and Drug Administration for women with severe

IBS and diarrhea (Figure 8-4). This drug is absolutely not to be used if your bowel pattern switches between diarrhea and constipation or if you are constipated. This is an excellent drug in terms of benefits for IBS and diarrhea[1,2,6] (Figure 8-4). It also improves well-being in people with IBS. While the drug clearly works for IBS with diarrhea, it can have very serious side effects, and the risk-to-benefit ratio has to be carefully weighed by you and your physician.

Constipation is a common side effect of alosetron use. In about 1 in 1,000 patients, serious complications can occur from constipation, including rarely deaths from bowel blockage and tearing (perforation). A problem with the blood supply to the colon, causing diarrhea with blood, a condition called ischemic colitis, occurs in about 1 in 250 people taking the drug. Recent reports suggest that people with IBS develop ischemic colitis more often than do people who are not suffering with IBS (the

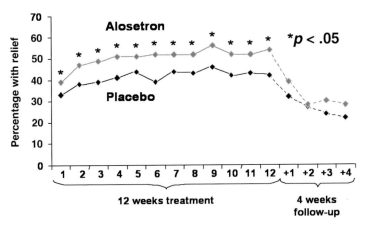

Figure 8-4: Results of a randomized double-blind placebo-controlled trial of alosetron in women with diarrhea and irritable bowel syndrome (IBS). Alosetron beat placebo in this study (p< .05 means a statistically significant result). Reproduced with permission from Camilleri M, Northcutt AR, Kong S, et al. Efficacy and safety of alosetron in women with irritable bowel syndrome: a randomised, placebo-controlled trial. Lancet 2000;355:1035–40.

risk is two to four times higher, but it is still rare).[7] However, alosetron clearly increases the risk of this problem.

Alosetron is definitely a useful agent for women with very severe IBS and diarrhea, but the drug is currently limited to only this group. People taking this drug need to be monitored by their doctors regularly. If you want to take the drug, you need to understand the serious side effects, sign a Patient-Physician Agreement with your physician, and carefully follow all directions.

Another drug that seems useful in IBS with diarrhea is cilansetron, but it can also cause ischemic colitis. This drug appears to work in both men and women and may be on the market one day.

AN OVERALL MANAGEMENT PLAN

As you can see, a number of different medications that can help with IBS are available, but the response to them is somewhat variable. Furthermore, only certain people will respond to certain types of medications, which makes this all very complicated. Many doctors divide IBS patients into two major categories, namely, those with mainly diarrhea and those with mainly constipation. Of course, many people change from diarrhea to constipation and back again, and some people only have minor bowel symptoms, which makes this distinction somewhat artificial. Still, it is a useful framework for thinking about the kinds of treatments to use for IBS.

I always start off recommending dietary management. This is so important because it is safe and can make a difference for life. I also liberally use fiber supplements (especially psyllium products) initially. Remember, dietary change and fiber supplements take time to work, and you need to allow a sufficient amount of time for benefits to be seen; it is not a "quick fix" approach. Fiber products can help constipation; sometimes diarrhea also improves as the stools firm up.

Medications you are taking for other problems need to be reviewed. Constipation and diarrhea can occur with many medications, and stopping them (if possible) will help. You should discuss all of your medications with your doctor. People are sometimes placed on medication regimens that are never stopped, even though the drugs aren't needed in the long term (especially if prescribed by a doctor elsewhere or if the person has no regular doctor); I've seen this quite often, especially with older people.

If constipation remains a problem despite dietary adjustment, then adding a safe and gentle laxative such as one of the osmotic laxatives is a very reasonable next step unless this has already failed. Next, it is reasonable to try tegaserod (Zelnorm), which will work for approximately two-thirds of patients. The main disadvantage of tegaserod is that when the treatment is stopped, the symptoms will come back in many cases, which means that you need to continue taking the medication to keep the symptoms under control. Clearly, if you can get away with it, just dietary adjustment is preferable to taking any kind of drug for the long term. The same disadvantage applies to laxatives, which would also need to be taken for the long term in this situation.

Constipation can be very troubling. It is important to discuss with your physician the possibility that the constipation might be due to some kind of pelvic muscle problem that is blocking the normal passage of stool. Biofeedback can be very effective for treating this type of constipation; about 75% of patients get better with this muscle re-training, so it is important to consider although how long the benefit lasts is less clear.

If diarrhea is the major problem and if fiber supplements don't firm up the stool enough, I like to add loperamide (Imodium) to the patient's regimen to prevent the diarrhea rather than prescribing it after the diarrhea occurs. Sometimes, high doses are needed, but this medicine can be very helpful for many people and appears to be particularly safe.

Antidepressant medications are very useful for pain and also can influence the bowel disturbance in a positive way if used properly. The tricyclic antidepressants, in particular, are helpful if diarrhea is a problem because they have a constipating effect. On the other hand, selective serotonin reuptake inhibitors such as fluoxetine (Prozac) tend to be more helpful if constipation is the problem as they have a tendency to induce diarrhea. Of course, even some people with diarrhea will do very well on fluoxetine, and some people with constipation will do very well on the tricyclics. The dosage and the individual drug chosen can be important in influencing what works well or not at all.

Psychological treatments can help too; discuss this issue with your doctor. Seek advice from your doctor on alternative treatments as well. If your pain is severe and constant, ask your doctor about a referral to a specialty pain clinic. Injection of the muscles of the abdomen with a local anesthetic and a steroid can sometimes relieve muscle pain that can be confused with IBS.

You need to work with your doctor when it comes to creating a management plan for IBS. Much of it will be up to you in terms of adjusting diet through trial and error and in terms of when medication is taken and what will work best for you. There is a wide variation in the response to treatment, which makes it more difficult for your doctor unless you provide accurate feedback about what is happening with your treatment so that logical changes can be made. On the other hand, I know that the vast majority of people with IBS who are properly managed and who work with their doctors achieve a substantial improvement in their symptoms, and some people actually virtually lose all of their symptoms.

Take-Home Messages

- Many drugs taken for irritable bowel syndrome (IBS) have not been scientifically established to help in IBS, but clinical experience with them suggests some benefits.
- Drugs used for IBS treatment are best taken for short periods to control exacerbations of symptoms.
- Antispasmodic drugs can relieve abdominal pain in IBS; they are best taken before pain occurs (such as before a meal).
- Antidiarrheal drugs such as loperamide (Imodium) help alleviate diarrhea but not pain or bloating in IBS; take them before diarrhea starts if you can.
- Antidepressants seem to have a specific bowel benefit in IBS. They can be very helpful for some people but for maximal benefit require the physician to be experienced in using them for this purpose. They take weeks to work, not days, and they can cause serious side effects.
- Tegaserod (Zelnorm) works better than placebo for women with IBS and constipation.
- Alosetron (Lotronex) works better than placebo in women with IBS and diarrhea. Side effects limit its use, however.

CHAPTER 9

THE FUTURE, AND WHERE TO SEEK MORE HELP

"I never think of the future—it comes soon enough." (Albert Einstein, 1879–1955)

"The future ain't what it used to be." (Yogi Berra, 1925–)

Much research into irritable bowel disease (IBS) is now ongoing, but more is needed. Indeed, it has been a struggle to convince the National Institutes of Health in the United States that IBS is an important enough problem to be funded adequately although this situation has begun to change. Fundamental research into the underlying causes of IBS hold the most hope for identifying real cures. For example, if inflammation is of primary importance, then attacking this problem may lead to long-term benefits. Furthermore, although not possible now, in the future it may be feasible to prevent the development of IBS after an attack of gastroenteritis. So what might be around the corner?

PROBIOTICS

We all have bowel bacteria, and loads of them. It has been theorized that changing the bowel bacteria might help in IBS, but to do this is difficult. Probiotics are live or dead bacteria that are administered in the hope of changing the bacteria in the bowel for the better. There is a lot of interest in this area, and much research is ongoing to understand the role of these products. You can buy lots of different probiotics at a health food store or pharmacy, but what will really work for a person with IBS is much less certain. Whether the bacteria in probiotics are alive or dead, the number of bacteria, the mix of bacteria, and how the bacteria are delivered are all likely to affect the benefits of this treatment. However, there have been some promising early results,[1] and it may be that

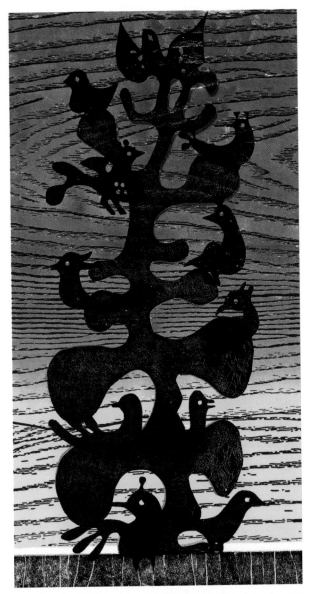

And what will the dawn bring, from the International Foundation for Functional Gastrointestinal Disorders (IFFGD) Art of IBS Collection. Printed with permission from the IFFGD (© 2004 IFFGD).

this becomes prime time for IBS in the near future. For example, VSL#3, a patented *Lactobacillus* preparation, helped bloating but not other symptoms in one trial.[2]

The informed "IBS consumer" will need to look very carefully at the evidence (when it appears) for the benefit of this type of treatment, using those principles of evidence-based medicine that are discussed in this book (see page 68).

ANTIBIOTICS

Antibiotics can also change bowel bacteria, at least for a short time. The role of antibiotics in IBS treatment is unclear but may be more important than was once suspected.[3] However, it is not practical to take antibiotics for a long period in most situations; indeed, which antibiotics will really work (assuming any will) remains uncertain. The preliminary evidence now available may lead to some advances, however, so you should watch for developments in regard to antibiotic therapy.

FECAL TRANSPLANTATION

"Some remedies are worse than the disease." (Publius Syrius, first century BC)

Some rather unusual approaches to the potential treatment of IBS have been proposed. One suggestion is that because the bacteria in the bowel may be abnormal in IBS, the transplantation of bacteria from other people might be helpful. Some claim that this treatment does help the symptoms of IBS, but this has not been shown in proper randomized placebo-controlled studies. Furthermore, it is likely that any transplanted bacteria are quickly eliminated, and the potential dangers of this approach remain somewhat unclear. Although the concept of altering the bacterial flora in the bowel is an attractive consideration, I certainly do not suggest the fecal transplant approach. In summary, some brave souls have had fecal transplants for their bowel problems; this is not recommended!

NEW DRUGS THAT BLOCK PAIN OR DISCOMFORT

Several drugs that are currently either in development or in testing for IBS may help with the pain or discomfort of IBS.[4,5] For example, certain opioids agonists (kappa agonists), which block pain receptors on pain fibers and which are not addictive, are now being tested for use in IBS treatment. Some of these look promising in small studies but large trials are not available. Another group of agents of potential value are the tachykinin receptor antagonists, which block pain receptors of a different class.[4,5] These drugs can be constipating and may therefore be of most benefit for people with diarrheal IBS. Yet another group of agents are the corticotropin-releasing factor (CRF) antagonists. (CRF was discussed previously in relation to its potential importance in mediating the stress response; see page 63.) Only a few of these compounds are currently available, but more may be developed and tested in people. Some believe that pain-blocking drugs will be one of the most potent new approaches to treating IBS, but we will just have to wait and see.

NEW SEROTONIN AGENTS

Chapter 8 outlined the value of agents (such as alosetron, a serotonin type-3 receptor antagonist) that affect the serotonin receptor. Another serotonin type-3 receptor antagonist is cilansetron.[5] It appears to work not only in women but also in men and has promise in the treatment of diarrheal IBS. However, it may also have a side-effect profile that is similar to that of alosetron.

OTHER NEW TREATMENTS ON THE HORIZON

Drugs that affect the sympathetic or parasympathetic nervous system have been considered in IBS treatment and may hold some promise. Clonidine (Catapres) is available for the treatment of high blood pressure. This drug works on the autonomic nervous system (through the α_2-adrenergic receptor) and has been shown to reduce pain sensation from the bowel in people with IBS.[6] It also helps with diarrhea and urgency. However, clonidine also lowers blood pressure and can therefore cause some side effects; at present, determining the correct dose is rather difficult. A number of similar agents that are in development may have some role in IBS treatment in the future. Other drug companies are working on developing new drugs that will directly or indirectly relax smooth muscle and therefore be of benefit in managing the pain of IBS.

There is also a family of compounds that actually help nerve cells regenerate and reconnect in the bowel, which may hold great hope not only for people with IBS but also for those with other serious nerve diseases of the bowel.[5] One such compound is called recombinant human brain-derived neurotrophic factor; another is called recombinant human neurotrophic factor 3. Both of these have entered some human trials on constipation, and this work is being watched with great interest.

A number of other drugs that either stimulate or antagonize other important neurotransmitter receptors in the bowel are in development.[5] Again, whether any of these drugs will become available to help people with IBS is not known at this stage. Many compounds come and go without ever reaching clinical practice because of toxicity, a lack of any benefit, or both. Only a very small number of drugs get through the testing process. When new drugs do become available, however, it is hoped that you will be in a position to be able to judge whether or not those drugs are right for you. Just because a drug is on the market and advertised on TV, don't fall into the trap of believing that this means it must be really safe. A good example of this is the arthritis drug Vioxx; widely used and aggressively advertised in the media, it was a good drug that caused fewer stomach ulcers (and deaths from ulcer complications like bleeding), but unfortunately, it also increased the risk of heart attacks.

Genetics seems likely to be a tool that will be used in the future to help guide how best to treat IBS (and many other medical conditions). I am convinced that this field, called pharmacogenomics, will grow greatly in the twenty-first century. Already, some of the genes that influence the response to alosetron (Lotronex) have been identified although the findings are not yet ready for practical use.[7]

Another approach has been to try stimulating the bowel electrically. This methodology has a long way to go but may be of help in the near future.

You may want to volunteer for a study of new IBS treatments. Many large centers such as the Mayo Clinic, the University of California in Los Angeles, and the University of North Carolina conduct such trials regularly. The pharmaceutical industry often conducts countrywide studies. Local and national medical organizations can put you in touch with the latest trials.

WHERE TO SEEK MORE HELP

There is help out there, and you may need to seek it out. The rest of this chapter summarizes some of the available support structures. Being proactive here can help you.

Patient Support Groups and Organizations
International Foundation for Functional Gastrointestinal Disorders. The International Foundation for Gastrointestinal Disorders was founded by Nancy Norton and is the best-known national organization in this field. It offers lifetime or yearly membership, an excellent magazine that is very informative, and the opportunity to meet with people who are also suffering with similar symptoms. The organization includes prominent experts on its board (this author is a board mem-

ber). Nancy has been particularly active and successful in increasing the funding for studies of IBS and related disorders. This organization is very worthy of your interest and support if you suffer with IBS or if friends or family members are so afflicted. It can be contacted through the following address, telephone number, and Web site:

International Foundation for Functional Gastrointestinal Disorders
P. O. Box 17864
Milwaukee, WI 53217
Telephone: 888-964-2001 (toll free)
<http://www.iffgd.org>

Medical and Government Organizations
- American College of Gastroenterology (<http://www.acg.gi.org>)
- American Dietetic Association (<http://www.eatright.org>)
- American Gastroenterological Association (<http://www. gastro.org>)
- Centers for Disease Control and Prevention (<http://www.cdc.gov>)
- Mayo Clinic Health Information (<http://www.MayoClinic.com>)
- National Digestive Disease Information Clearinghouse (<http://www.digestive.niddk.nih.gov>) (Look here for clinical trials of new treatments for IBS.)
- Rome Foundation (<http://www.romecriteria.org>)

Medical Journals
Many scientific medical journals publish articles on IBS that may be of interest. Look for peer-reviewed journals, which means that before publication, the articles must pass muster after

being critically examined by experts in the field. However, do not blindly believe a study's conclusion; it could still be wrong!

There are many medical journals, but the following are the top journals whose articles you might want to consult and discuss with your doctor:

- *Annals of Internal Medicine* (<http://www.annals.org>)
- *British Medical Journal* (<http://www.bmj.com>) (free on the Web for all, and an excellent source)
- *Lancet* (<http://www.thelancet.com>)
- *New England Journal of Medicine* (<http://www.content.nejm.org>)
- *American Journal of Gastroenterology* (<http://www.amjgastro.com>)
- *Gastroenterology* (<http://www.gastrojournal.org>)
- *Gut* (<http://www.bowel.bmjjournals.com>)

To guide your understanding, look particularly for meta-analyses or review articles on IBS treatment.

Books

The Functional Gastrointestinal Disorders[8] is an excellent and authoritative resource for doctors; patients may also find much of interest in it. It is written by the world's authorities in the field and edited by this author, among others.

There are other books that give advice, but remember to try and decide whether what you are reading is evidence based or not. Many of the opinions will be wrong!

The Internet

Be cautious! Much misinformation is out there, so always apply the principles of evidence-based medicine you have learned from this book. Testimonials do not prove that a treatment works! Indeed, you usually don't find negative testimonials, but no treatment will work for everyone, so you cannot be getting the full truth. Before you follow any advice, make sure it is safe, at least; seek the opinion of your physician if there is any doubt.

Literature searches can be conducted with *PubMed* (<http://www.ncbi.nim.gov>), a free and excellent resource on the Internet. If you enter "IBS" or "irritable bowel syndrome," a list of many articles in peer-reviewed and nonpeer-reviewed journals will appear, most with short summaries (abstracts). Some complete articles are available free on the Internet whereas others can be purchased for a small fee. Even though you can retrieve many articles with this great tool, it does not identify all relevant medical articles, which requires use of various search engines, careful consideration of search terms, and manual searching of reference lists found in the major articles.

FUNCTIONAL GASTROINTESTINAL DISORDERS

A. Esophageal Disorders

A1. Globus

A2. Rumination syndrome

A3. Functional chest pain of presumed esophageal origin

A4. Functional heartburn

A5. Functional dysphagia

A6. Unspecific functional esophageal disorder

B. Gastroduodenal Disorders

B1. Functional dyspepsia

    B1a. Ulcer-like dyspepsia

    B1b. Dysmotility-like dyspepsia

    B1c. Unspecified (nonspecific) dyspepsia

B2. Aerophagia

B3. Functional vomiting

C. Bowel Disorders

C1. Irritable bowel syndrome

    C1a. Constipation predominant

    C1b. Diarrhea predominant

    C1c. Alternating constipation and diarrhea

C2. Functional abdominal bloating

C3. Functional constipation

C4. Functional diarrhea

C5. Unspecified functional bowel disorder

D. Functional Abdominal Pain

D1. Functional abdominal pain syndrome

D2. Unspecified functional abdominal pain

E. Functional Disorders of the Biliary Tract and Pancreas

E1. Gallbladder dysfunction

E2. Sphincter of Oddi dysfunction

Continued on next page

F.   Anorectal Disorders

F1.   Functional fecal incontinence

F2.   Functional anorectal pain

   F2a. Levator ani syndrome

   F2b. Proctalgia fugax

F3.   Pelvic-floor dyssynergia

G.   Functional Pediatric Disorders

G1.   Vomiting

   G1a. Infant regurgitation

   G1b. Infant rumination syndrome

   G1c. Cyclic vomiting syndrome

G2.   Abdominal pain

   G2a. Functional dyspepsia

      G2a1. Ulcer-like dyspepsia

      G2a2. Dysmotility-like dyspepsia

      G2a3. Unspecified (nonspecific) dyspepsia

   G2b. Irritable bowel syndrome

   G2c. Functional abdominal pain

   G2d. Abdominal migraine

   G2e. Aerophagia

G3.   Functional diarrhea

G4.   Disorders of defecation

   G4a. Infant dyschezia

   G4b. Functional constipation

   G4c. Functional fecal retention

   G4d. Functional nonretentive fecal soiling

QUESTIONNAIRE FOR FUNCTIONAL BOWEL DISORDERS

1. In the last 3 months, did you *often*★ have discomfort or pain in you abdomen (tummy)?
   - ❑ No or rarely
   - ❑ Yes

2. Does your discomfort or pain often get better or stop after you have a bowel movement?
   - ❑ No or rarely
   - ❑ Yes

3. When the discomfort or pain starts, do you often have a change in your usual number of bowel movements (either more or fewer)?
   - ❑ No or rarely
   - ❑ Yes

4. When the discomfort or pain starts, do you often have either softer or harder stools than usual?
   - ❑ No or rarely
   - ❑ Yes

5. Have you had any of the following symptoms at least one-fourth (1/4) of the time (occasions or days) in the last 3 months? (check all that apply)
   - ❑ Fewer than three bowel movements a week (0-2)
   - ❑ More than three bowel movements a day (4 or more)
   - ❑ Hard or lumpy stools
   - ❑ Loose, mushy, or watery stools
   - ❑ Straining during a bowel movement
   - ❑ Having to rush to the toilet to have a bowel movement
   - ❑ Feeling of incomplete emptying after a bowel movement
   - ❑ Passing of mucus (slime) during a bowel movement
   - ❑ Abdominal fullness, bloating, or swelling
   - ❑ A sensation that the stool cannot be passed (ie,blocked) when having a bowel movement
   - ❑ A need to press on or around your anus or vagina to try to remove stool in order to complete the bowel movement

6. In the last 3 months, did you have loose, mushy, or watery stools during more than three quarters (3/4) of your bowel movements?
   - ❑ No or rarely
   - ❑ Yes

★*Often* means that the symptoms were present during at least 3 weeks (at least 1 day in each week) in the last 3 months.

If you answered YES to question 1 and YES to any of the other questions, you may have IBS or another functional bowel disorder. You should consult your doctor for evaluation and treatment.

Adapted from Doug Drossman, MD, with permission.

abdomen   The area of the body below the chest; may be referred to as the tummy or stomach; contains the intestinal organs.

abdominal distention   The feeling that the abdomen is swollen or bloated. The swelling may be visible to you; you may look pregnant, and others may be able to see the swelling.

abuse   Threats or actions of a sexual, physical, verbal, or emotional type. Usually, there is a difference in power between the abuser and the victim.

aerophagia   Swallowing of air; usually associated with repeated belching (burping) because belching makes one swallow more air without knowing it.

afferent nerve   A nerve that carries sensations to the brain from an organ such as the stomach or large or small bowel.

alarm symptoms   Worrying symptoms such as unexplained weight loss, repeated vomiting, blood in the stool, trouble swallowing, or fever. These symptoms are not explained by irritable bowel syndrome but must have another explanation; thus, people with these symptoms should see their physician promptly. (Also called "red flags" in the medical literature.)

antidepressants   A group of drugs that change neurotransmitters in the brain, such as the chemical serotonin. These drugs are used to treat depression but also are useful in the management of irritable bowel syndrome, not because they act on depression but because they reduce pain processing both in the brain and in the bowel.

anal fissure   A crack in the skin near the anus; it causes itching or pain, particularly when opening the bowels, and can occur with constipation (hard stools crack the skin on straining).

anorexia   Loss of appetite or lack of desire for food.

anxiety   A sense of feeling nervous or worried that often occurs with other symptoms such as excessive fear, churning in the abdomen, shortness of breath, a "racing heart," and sweating.

belching   The bringing up (burping) of air from the stomach through the mouth (usually air that has been swallowed).

biofeedback The use of an electronic or other device that gives information by either sound or vision so that an individual can be taught to control a process. A person with constipation can use biofeedback to unlearn the tensing of the muscles that prevents the normal passing of stool.

blind Said of a clinical trial in which the patients are unaware of the treatment and in which those administering the treatment are also unaware of what is being given (called "double blinding").

bloating A feeling of fullness or distention that either may be just felt or may actually be visible (visible abdominal distension).

Bristol stool form scale A seven-point scale that rates the stool from watery to hard or lumpy, developed in Bristol, England. The numbers on the scale correspond reasonably well to the measurement (with objective tests) of movement of material through the bowel.

bulking agents Drugs that increase the amount of stool and help soften the stool because increased water is bound to it. Bulking agents of plant origin include bran. Bulking agents cannot be split by the usual enzymes in the human bowel but may be partially digested in the colon, producing excessive gas.

cholecystokinin (CCK) A hormone that is released from the small bowel in response to a meal; also a neurotransmitter substance in the nerves in the bowel.

cognitive behavior therapy In terms of irritable bowel syndrome, a therapy that explores how certain thoughts and behaviors may negatively upset the bowel so that they can be modified to help the patient cope with symptoms; it is a useful for learning how to cope with irritable bowel syndrome and may help reduce the symptoms.

colic Pain or cramps that come and go, usually over minutes.

colon The large bowel, connecting the anus to the small bowel.

corticotropin-releasing factor (CRF) A stress hormone released from the brain.

control In a trial, someone who does not receive the active treatment but usually receives a placebo (dummy) instead.

depression A feeling of sadness, tearfulness, and pessimism that can vary from mild to severe. Appetite is usually suppressed, and the sleep pattern is upset. There is often fatigue and loss of energy. There may be feelings of guilt and worthlessness. In severe types, there are suicidal feelings.

dietary fiber   Naturally occurring plant materials that cannot be normally digested in the small bowel and that therefore increase stool weight and soften stool.

discomfort   A feeling that is not painful but is unpleasant.

distention of the abdomen   A swelling of the stomach or abdomen that can be seen by either oneself or another observer.

double blind   Said of a therapeutic experiment in which neither those participating in the experiment nor those conducting the experiment know what type of therapy is actually being given.

dyspepsia   A feeling of pain or discomfort in the upper stomach area.

early satiety   Inability to finish eating a normal meal because of discomfort; this can be due to stomach dysfunction. Also called "early satiation."

efferent nerve   Nerve fibers that carry impulses from the brain or spinal cord, which lead to a muscle to contract.

enteric nervous system   A complex system of nerves that works automatically within the walls of the bowel and does not require the brain in order to function effectively.

esophagus   The swallowing tube connecting the back of the mouth (pharynx) to the stomach.

fart   The passage of gas (wind) through the anus, or the sound, smell, or odor of gas passing through this area.

flatulence   A vague term that may mean the passing of gas through the anus or any type of feeling of bloating or gaseousness.

flatus   Passage of gas through the anus.

functional bowel disorder   A disorder that can occur in the upper or lower abdominal area and for which no clear-cut cause can be found when the bowel is examined by radiography or endoscopy.

gas   Gas escaping from the mouth or the anus; called "wind" in England and Australia.

gastrin   A hormone that is released from the stomach and stimulates acid secretion.

gastroenterologist   A physician specialist with a major interest and expertise in the gastrointestinal (bowel) system.

gastroesophageal reflux   The passage of stomach contents into the swallowing tube (esophagus), typically causing heartburn (from stomach acid in the wrong place).

gut hypersensitivity   Unusual sensitivity of the bowel to normal or abnormal stimuli (such as the inflation of a balloon within the bowel).

heartburn   A burning sensation or discomfort in the chest, usually rising up toward the throat and typically temporarily relieved with an antacid.

Helicobacter pylori   A bacterium that causes a stomach infection that always causes inflammation. The infection is usually acquired in childhood and persists for life. Although the infection can cause chronic peptic ulcers and gastric cancer, most people with the infection do not become ill from it. It does not cause irritable bowel syndrome.

5-hydroxytryptamine (5-HT)   One of the key bowel neurotransmitters; it is also an important neurotransmitter in the brain. Also called serotonin.

hypnotherapy   The application of hypnosis (a state of heightened suggestibility and deep relaxation) to treat symptoms. It does seem to help some sufferers with irritable bowel syndrome.

incontinence of feces   The leakage of stool (liquid or solid) into the underwear. This may occur with or without a sense of needing to defecate. It can be due to muscle or nerve damage around the anus.

indigestion   A vague term that can mean pain or discomfort in the stomach area, heartburn, passage of excessive gas through the mouth, or many other symptoms.

irritable bowel syndrome (IBS)   An important and common disease that causes abdominal discomfort or pain associated with abnormal bowel movements (either constipation or diarrhea) and often bloating or visible abdominal swelling.

laxative   A drug that increases stool frequency or induces looser or more watery stools by a number of different mechanisms.

Manning Criteria   A set of criteria described by Dr. Manning and colleagues in an important medical paper that showed that certain symptoms could distinguish irritable bowel syndrome patients from those with other bowel diseases.

meta-analysis A method for accurately combining data from randomized controlled trials so that the overall effect of a treatment can be estimated. Meta-analysis of randomized trials represents a good way to assess the evidence of the benefit of a treatment.

nausea A feeling of the need to vomit; a queasiness or feeling of being sick.

neurotransmitter A substance that is released from nerve cells and that allows the nerve cells to talk to each other and transmit signals accurately. Serotonin (5-HT) is one important neurotransmitter.

off label Describes the way medications are appropriately used by physicians even though the US Food and Drug Administration has not specifically approved them for a particular use.

pain An unpleasant sensation that may feel as if tissue damage is occurring. It may not be possible to accurately distinguish pain from discomfort (although in some cultures, the distinction is clearer than in others).

parasympathetic nervous system Part of the autonomic nervous system from the brain that controls the bowel and other bodily functions.

peptic ulcer A large hole in the lining of the stomach or upper small intestine (duodenum). The common underlying causes are *Helicobacter pybri* and aspirin or arthritis drugs. Acid reduction can heal the ulcer.

placebo A dummy or inactive treatment ("sugar pill").

placebo response The response to dummy or inert treatment in a randomized controlled trial.

primary care First-contact doctor care, in which patients can see a physician without referral by another doctor. Also called "general practice" in some countries.

probiotic A type of medicine that changes the bowel bacteria to make its composition healthier by introducing live or dead organisms that alter the bowel bacteria.

proctalgia fugax Sharp, often severe, but short-lived pain in the anal area, due to muscle spasm.

prokinetic A drug that enhances the speed of material being moved through the bowel by acting at the level of the nervous system, usually in the bowel, leading to a release of neurotransmitters.

psychology A science that deals with mental processes and the mind.

psychiatric diagnosis   The diagnosis of a disease (as classified by a psychiatrist) that includes depression and anxiety. However, one may have feelings of depression or anxiety and not have a psychiatric diagnosis of anxiety or depression.

psychiatrist   A medical doctor specializing in mental health problems.

psychologist   A nonmedical specialist (usually with a master's or doctoral [PhD] degree) who treats problems of the mind and mental processes.

psychosomatic   An old term that describes diseases that were thought to be due to psychological characteristics. For example, peptic ulcer used to be called a psychosomatic disease until it was realized that most peptic ulcers are caused by an infection, *Helicobacter pylori*.

quality of life   The feeling of well-being, both physical and psychological, that can be affected by disease or illness.

randomization   The process by which subjects in a clinical trial are selected (not by the investigator but usually by a computer) in random order so that people being treated and people not being treated are similar, making the study more likely to provide a true result.

Rome criteria   The international diagnostic criteria (ie, a list of symptoms) for irritable bowel syndrome and other functional bowel disorders, created by a consensus of experts.

small bowel   The bowel connecting the stomach to the colon. It is about 30 feet in length and is key in the absorption of food.

stress   Any external or internal factor that interferes with a person's life, including health.

stool   Digestive waste that is stored and passed by the colon to the anus.

transit time (bowel)   The time it takes for food or other material to move through a specified region of the bowel.

visceral hypersensitivity   An increased intestinal sensitivity to various stimuli (such as the inflation of a balloon in the bowel).

vomiting   The violent expulsion of stomach contents through the mouth.

REFERENCES

These are cited by author, article title, journal title, year published, volume number, and page numbers.

CHAPTER 1

1. Thompson WG, Heaton K. Functional bowel disorders in apparently healthy people. Gastroenterology 1980;79:283–8.

2. Talley NJ, Weaver AL, Zinsmeister AR, Melton LJ 3rd. Onset and disappearance of gastrointestinal symptoms and functional gastrointestinal disorders. Am J Epidemiol 1992;136:165–77.

3. Talley NJ, Zinsmeister AR, Melton LJ 3rd. Irritable bowel syndrome in a community: symptom subgroups, risk factors, and health care utilization. Am J Epidemiol 1995;142:76–83.

4. Marshall BJ. The 1995 Albert Lasker Medical Research Award. *Helicobacter pylori*. The etiologic agent for peptic ulcer. JAMA 1995;274:1064–6.

5. Talley NJ, Gabriel SE, Harmsen WS, et al. Medical costs in community subjects with irritable bowel syndrome. Gastroenterology 1995;109:1736–41.

CHAPTER 2

1. Drossman DA, Li Z, Andruzzi E, et al. U. S. householder survey of functional gastrointestinal disorders. Prevalence, sociodemography, and health impact. Dig Dis Sci 1993;38:1569–80.

2. Whitehead WE, Winget C, Fedoravicius AS, et al. Learned illness behavior in patients with irritable bowel syndrome and peptic ulcer. Dig Dis Sci 1982;27:202–8.

3. Cash BD, Schoenfeld P, Chey WD. The utility of diagnostic tests in irritable bowel syndrome patients: a systematic review. Am J Gastroenterol 2002;97:2812–9.

4. Degen LP, Phillips SF. How well does stool form reflect colonic transit? Gut 1996;39:109–13.

5. Aichbichler BW, Wenzl HH, Santa Ana CA, et al. A comparison of stool characteristics from normal and constipated people. Dig Dis Sci 1998;43:2353–62.

6. Lewis MJ, Reilly B, Houghton LA, Whorwell PJ. Ambulatory abdominal inductance plethysmography: towards objective assessment of abdominal distension in irritable bowel syndrome. Gut 2001;48:216–20.

7. Manning AP, Thompson WG, Heaton KW, Morris AF. Towards positive diagnosis of the irritable bowel. Br Med J 1978;2:653–4.

8. Powell R. On certain painful afflictions of the intestinal canal. Medical Transcripts Royal College of Physicians 1818;6:106–17.

9. Cumming W. Electro-galvanism in a peculiar affliction of the mucous membrane of the bowels. London Medical Gazette 1849;NS9:969–73.

10. Talley NJ. Dyspepsia and non-ulcer dyspepsia: an historical perspective. Med J Aust 1985;145:614–8.

CHAPTER 3

1. Locke GR III, Zinsmeister AR, Talley NJ, et al. Familial association in adults with functional gastrointestinal disorders. Mayo Clin Proc 2000;75:907–12.

2. Morris-Yates A, Talley NJ, Boyce PM, et al. Evidence of a genetic contribution to functional bowel disorder. Am J Gastroenterol 1998;93:1311–7.

3. Levy RL, Jones KR, Whitehead WE, et al. Irritable bowel syndrome in twins: heredity and social learning both contribute to etiology. Gastroenterology 2001;121:799–804.

4. Holtmann G, Siffert W, Haag S, et al. G-protein β 3 subunit 825 CC genotype is associated with unexplained (functional) dyspepsia. Gastroenterology 2004;126:971–79.

5. Gonsalkorale WM, Perrey C, Pravica K, et al. Interleukin 10 genotypes in irritable bowel syndrome: evidence for an inflammatory component? Gut 2003;52:91–3.

6. Yeo A, Boyd P, Lumsden S, et al. Association between a functional polymorphism in the serotonin transporter gene and diarrhoea predominant in irritable bowel syndrome in women. Gut 2004;53:1452–8.

7. Kim HJ, Camilleri M, Carlson PJ, et al. Association of distinct alpha(2) adrenoreceptor and serotinin transporter polymorphisms with constipation and somatic symptoms in functional gastrointestinal disorders. Gut 2004;53:829–37.

8. Chaudhary NA, Truelove SC. The irritable colon syndrome. A study of the clinical features, predisposing causes, and prognosis in 130 cases. QJM 1962;31:307–22.

9. Spiller RC. Postinfectious irritable bowel syndrome. Gastroenterology 2003;124:1662–71.

10. Talley NJ, Spiller R. Irritable bowel syndrome: a little understood organic bowel disease? Lancet 2002;360:555–64.

11. Chang L, Berman S, Mayer EA, et al. Brain responses to visceral and somatic stimuli in patients with irritable bowel syndrome with and without fibromyalgia. Am J Gastroenterol 2003;98:1354–61.

12. Naliboff BD, Berman S, Chang L, et al. Sex-related differences in IBS patients: central processing of visceral stimuli. Gastroenterology 2003;124:1738–47.

13. Naliboff BD, Derbyshire SW, Munakata J, et al. Cerebral activation in patients with irritable bowel syndrome and control subjects during rectosigmoid stimulation. Psychosom Med 2001;63:365–75.

14. Drossman DA, Talley NJ, Leserman J, et al. Sexual and physical abuse and gastrointestinal illness. Review and recommendations. Ann Intern Med 1995;123:782–94.

15. Talley NJ, Fett SL, Zinsmeister AR, Melton LJ III. Gastrointestinal tract symptoms and self-reported abuse: a population-based study. Gastroenterology 1994;107:1040–9.

16. Bouin M, Plourde V, Boivin M, et al. Rectal distention testing in patients with irritable bowel syndrome: sensitivity, specificity, and predictive values of pain sensory thresholds. Gastroenterology 2002;122:1771–7.

17. Mertz H, Naliboff B, Munakata J, et al. Altered rectal perception is a biological marker of patients with irritable bowel syndrome. Gastroenterology 1995;109:40–52.

18. Kellow JE, Phillips SF. Altered small bowel motility in irritable bowel syndrome is correlated with symptoms. Gastroenterology 1987;92:1885–93.

19. Chey WY, Jin HO, Lee MH, et al. Colonic motility abnormality in patients with irritable bowel syndrome exhibiting abdominal pain and diarrhea. Am J Gastroenterol 2001;96:1499–506.

20. Lee OY, Mayer EA, Schmulson M, et al. Gender-related differences in IBS symptoms. Am J Gastroenterol 2001;96:2184–93.

CHAPTER 4

1. Thompson WG. Placebos: a review of the placebo response. Am J Gastroenterol 2000;95:1637–43.

2. Blackwell B, Bloomfield SS, Buncher CR. Demonstration to medical students of placebo responses and non-drug factors. Lancet 1972;1:1279–82.

3. Vase L, Robinson ME, Verne GN, Price DD. The contributions of suggestion, desire, and expectation to placebo effects in irritable bowel syndrome patients. An empirical investigation. Pain 2003;105:17–25.

4. Benedetti F. The opposite effects of the opiate antagonist naloxone and the cholecystokinin antagonist proglumide on placebo analgesia. Pain 1996;64:535–43.

5. Talley NJ. Unnecessary abdominal and back surgery in irritable bowel syndrome: time to stem the flood now? Gastroenterology 2004;126(7):1899–903.

6. Dans AL, Dans LF, Guyatt GH, Richardson S. Users' guides to the medical literature. XIV. How to decide on the applicability of clinical trial results to your patient. Evidence-Based Medicine Working Group. JAMA 1998;279:545–9.

7. Oxman AD, Sackett DL, Guyatt GH. Users' guides to the medical literature. I. How to get started. The Evidence-Based Medicine Working Group. JAMA 1993;270:2093–5.

8. Horton R. The lessons of MMR. Lancet 2004;363:747–9.

9. DiMasi JA, Hansen RW, Grabowski HG. The price of innovation: new estimates of drug development costs. J Health Econ 2003; 22:151–85.

CHAPTER 5

1. Talley NJ. Pharmacologic therapy for the irritable bowel syndrome. Am J Gastroenterol 2003;98:750–8.

2. Bijkerk CJ, Muris JWM, Knottnerus JA, et al. Systematic review: the role of different types of fibre in the treatment of irritable bowel syndrome. Aliment Pharmacol Ther 2004;19:245–52.

3. Atkinson W, Sheldon TA, Whorwell PJ, Shaath N. Food elimination based on IgG antibodies in irritable bowel syndrome: a randomized controlled trial. Gut 2004;53:1459–64.

4. Whorton J. Civilisation and the colon: constipation as the "disease of diseases." Br Med J 2000;321:1586–9.

5. Tjeerdsma HC, Smout AJ, Akkermans LM. Voluntary suppression of defecation delays gastric emptying. Dig Dis Sci 1993;38:832–6.

6. Heymen S, Jones KR, Scarlett Y, Whitehead WE. Biofeedback treatment of constipation: a critical review. Dis Colon Rectum 2003;46:1208–17.

CHAPTER 6

1. Yadav SK, Jain AK, Tripathi SN, Gupta JP. Irritable bowel syndrome: therapeutic evaluation of indigenous drugs. Indian J Med Res 1989;90:496–503.

2. Walker AF, Middleton RW, Petrowicz O. Artichoke leaf extract reduces symptoms of irritable bowel syndrome in a post-marketing surveillance study. Phytother Res 2001;15:58–61.

3. Bensoussan A, Talley NJ, Hing M, et al. Treatment of irritable bowel syndrome with Chinese herbal medicine. JAMA 1998; 280:1585–9.

4. Tovey P. A single-blind trial of reflexology for irritable bowel syndrome. Br J Gen Pract 2002;52:19–23.

5. Chan J, Carr I, Mayberry JF. The role of acupuncture in the treatment of irritable bowel syndrome: a pilot study. Hepato-gastroenterology 1997;44:1328–30.

6. Fireman Z, Segal A, Kopelman Y, et al. Acupuncture treatment for irritable bowel syndrome. A double-blind controlled study. Digestion 2001;64:100–3.

7. Rohrbock RB, Hammer J, Vogelsang H, et al. Acupuncture has a placebo effect on rectal perception but not on distensibility and spatial summation: a study in health and IBS. Am J Gastroenterol 2003;99:1990–7.

8. Vege SS, Locke GR III, Weaver AL, et al. Functional gastrointestinal disorders among people with sleep disturbances: a population-based study. Mayo Clin Proc 2004;79:1501–6.

9. Thompson JJ, Elsenbruch S, Harnish MJ, Orr WC. Autonomic functioning during REM sleep differentiates IBS symptom subgroups. Am J Gastroenterol 2002;97:3147–53.

10. Taneja I, Deepak KK, Pojary G, et al. Yogic versus conventional treatment in diarrhea-predominant irritable bowel syndrome: a randomized control study. Appl Psychophysiol Biofeedback 2004;29:19–33.

11. Pettinciti PM. Meditation, yoga, and guided imagery. Nur Clin North Am 2001;36:47–56.

12. Gonsalkorale WM, Miller V, Afzal A, Whorwell PJ. Long term benefits of hypnotherapy for irritable bowel syndrome. Gut 2003;52:1623–9.

13. Talley NJ, Owen BK, Boyce P, Paterson K. Psychological treatments for irritable bowel syndrome: a critique of controlled treatment trials. Am J Gastroenterol 1996;91:277–83.

14. Calvert EL, Houghton LA, Cooper P, et al. Long-term improvement in functional dyspepsia using hypnotherapy. Gastroenterology 2002;123:1778–85.

15. Boyce PM, Talley NJ, Balaam B, et al. A randomized controlled trial of cognitive behavior therapy, relaxation training, and routine clinical care for the irritable bowel syndrome. Am J Gastroenterol 2003;98:2209–18.

16. Drossman DA, Toner BB, Whitehead WE, et al. Cognitive-behavioral therapy versus education and desipramine versus placebo for moderate to severe functional bowel disorders. Gastroenterology 2003;125:19–31.

17. Lackner JM, Mesmer C, Morley S, et al. Psychological treatments for irritable bowel syndrome: a systematic review and meta-analysis. J Consult Clin Psychol 2004;72:1100–13.

CHAPTER 7

1. Jones MP, Talley NJ, Nuyts G, Dubois D. Lack of objective evidence of efficacy of laxatives in chronic constipation. Dig Dis Sci 2002;47:2222–30.

2. Corazziari E, Badiali D, Habib FI, et al. Small volume isosmotic polyethylene glycol electrolyte balanced solution (PMF-100) in treatment of chronic nonorganic constipation. Dig Dis Sci 1996;41:1636–42.

3. Pittler MH, Ernst E. Peppermint oil for irritable bowel syndrome: a critical review and meta-analysis. Am J Gastroenterol 1998;93:1131–5.

4. Triadafilopoulos G, Tsang HP, Segall GM. Hot water swallows improve symptoms and accelerate esophageal clearance in esophageal motility disorders. J Clin Gastroenterol 1998; 26:239.

CHAPTER 8

1. Brandt LJ, Bjorkman D, Fennerty MB, et al. Systematic review on the management of irritable bowel syndrome in North America. Am J Gastroenterol 2002;97(11 Suppl):S7–26.

2. Lesbros-Pantoflickova D, Michetti P, Fried M, Blum AL. Meta-analysis: the treatment of irritable bowel syndrome. Aliment Pharmacol Ther 2004;20:1253–69.

3. Jackson JL, O'Malley PG, Tomkins G, et al. Treatment of functional gastrointestinal disorders with antidepressant medications: a meta-analysis. Am J Med 2000;108:65–72.

4. Ernst E. The risk-benefit profile of commonly used herbal therapies: ginkgo, St. John's wort, ginseng, *Echinacea*, saw palmetto, and kava. Ann Intern Med 2002;136:42–53.

5. Evans B, Clark W, Moore D, Whorwell PJ. Tegaserod for the treatment of irritable bowel syndrome. Cochrane Database Syst Rev 2004;1:CD003960.

6. Cremonini F, Delgado-Aros S, Camilleri M. Efficacy of alosetron in irritable bowel syndrome: a meta-analysis of randomized controlled trials. Neurogastroenterol Motil 2003;15:79–86.

7. Higgins PD, Davis KJ, Laine L. The epidemiology of ischaemic colitis. Aliment Pharmacol Ther 2004;19:729–38.

CHAPTER 9

1. Nobaek S, Johansson ML, Molin G, et al. Alteration of intestinal microflora is associated with reduction in abdominal bloating and pain in patients with irritable bowel syndrome. Am J Gastroenterol 2000;95:1231–8.

2. Kim HJ, Camilleri M, Mckinzie S, et al. A randomized controlled trial of a probiotic, VSL#3, on gut transit and symptoms in diarrhea-predominant irritable bowel syndrome. Aliment Pharmacol Ther 2003;17:895–904.

3. Pimentel M, Chow EJ, Lin HC. Normalization of lactulose breath testing correlates with symptom improvement in irritable bowel syndrome. A double-blind, randomized, placebo-controlled study. Am J Gastroenterol 2003;98:412–9.

4. Nam JH, Alnoah Z, Yerumula SR, Murthy S. Epidemiology, pathogenesis and treatment of irritable bowel syndrome. Expert Opin Ther Patents 2003;13:1213–67.

5. Talley NJ. Pharmacologic therapy for the irritable bowel syndrome. Am J Gastroenterol 2003;98:750–8.

6. Camilleri M, Kim DY, McKinzie S, et al. A randomized, controlled exploratory study of clonidine in diarrhea-predominant irritable bowel syndrome. Clin Gastroenterol Hepatol 2003;1:111–21.

7. Camilleri M, Atanasova E, Carlson PJ, et al. Serotonin-transporter polymorphism pharmacogenetics in diarrhea-predominant irritable bowel syndrome. Gastroenterology 2002;123:425–32.

8. Drossman DA et al, editors. The functional gastrointestinal disorders. Rome III. Degnon: 2006.

INDEX

Blacks, 82
   lactase deficiency, 99
Blinded, 71
Bloating, 135
Bloatometer, 32
Blood
   in stools, 27
Blood pressure
   high, 127
Books, 169
Bowels, 44. *See also* Large intes-
      tine
   abnormal contractions, 58
   abnormal sensation, 56–57
   biopsy samples, 52f
   bleeding, 27
   gas production in, 94–95
   regularity, 104–106
   short term changes in, 32
Brain, 45
   gastric emptying, 44
   MRI, 53
   PET, 53, 54f
   processing signals in, 52–53
Bran cereal, 89
Breakfast rush, 85
Bristol stool form scale, 31, 31f
Brody, Howard, 61
Brown rice, 89
Bulking agents, 92–93, 133–135
Burping
   reducing, 97–98

C
Caffeine, 120
Caffeine-containing drinks, 91
Calcium polycarbophil, 92
Campylobacter, 50

Cancer
   colon, 27, 87
Candy
   diet, 96
Carbohydrate absorption, 82
Catapres, 166
CCK. *See* Cholecystokinin
      (CCK)
Celiac disease, 36, 37
Cereal, 89, 105
Changjitai, 115
Charcoal
   activated, 142–143
Charcoal Plus, 142
CharcoCaps, 142
Child abuse, 54
Chinese herbal medicine, 115,
      116f, 118
Chlorophyll, 99
Cholecystokinin
   gallbladder, 58
Cholecystokinin (CCK), 46, 58
Cholestyramine (Questran Lite), 151
Cilansetron, 165
Cimetidine (Tagamet), 144
Citrucel, 92
Clinical trials, 72, 75, 76
   in humans, 75
Clonidine (Catapres), 166
Cochrane, Archie, 73
Cochrane Library, 73
Colace (dioctyl sodium sulfosuc-
      cinate), 136
Colitis
   mucous, 4
   spastic, 4
   ulcerative, 28

Colon, 44, 84
cancer, 27, 87
irrigation, 105
meridian, 119
transit
nuclear medicine test of,
155f
Colonoscopy, 28, 28f, 29
virtual, 37, 38f
Communist Party, 13
Complementary medicine,
113–114
Constipation, 7–8, 85, 89, 106,
110, 111
with alosetron, 157
biofeedback for, 159
drugs causing, 138
treatment, 98
Corn, 134
Correctol, 137
Corticotropin-releasing factor
(CRF), 45–46, 63, 165
Cost
of irritable bowel syndrome,
19–22
Cramps, 45
CRF. *See* Corticotropin-releasing
factor (CRF)
Crohn's disease, 28
Cumming, 34

D
Dairy products, 96
Deduction
method of, 69
Defecating proctography, 109
Depression, 127
Derifel, 99

Desipramine (Norpramin), 152
Diabetes, 127
Diagnosis, 32
Diarrhea, 7, 37, 45, 84
drugs causing, 138
first date, 1–2
traveler's, 32, 84
treatment of, 159
Diet
low-flatus, 98–99
sham, 103
Dietary fiber, 86–93
changing, 87
increasing, 88–92
Diet candy, 96
Diet drinks, 96
Digestive enzymes, 114
Dioctyl calcium sulfosuccinate,
136
Dioctyl sodium sulfosuccinate,
136
Diphenoxylate (Lomotil), 151
Discomfort
treatment of, 165
Doctors
financial relationships with
pharmaceutical compa-
nies, 78–79
Doteval, Gerhard, 34
Double blind, 71
Dried fruit, 89
Drinks
caffeine-containing, 91
diet, 96
Drossman, Doug, 34
Drugs
absorption of, 74–75
acid-reducing, 144–145

antidiarrheal, 139–142, 150–151
anxiety-reducing, 153
causing constipation, 138
discovery and development of,
    73–74
    treatment with, 73–77
gas-reducing, 142–143
names of, 77
research
    benefits and dangers, 77–80
side effects *vs.* allergies,
    145–148
Dulcolax, 137
Dumping syndrome, 43
Dyspepsia, 11
    functional, 12
    nonulcer, 12, 49, 131

E
Egyptian papyrus, 104
Elderly, 5, 27
Electrolytes, 84–85
    solution, 84
Electromyogram (EMG), 110
Emptying. *See* Gastric emptying
Endoscopy, 37
Enemas, 139
Enteric nervous system, 45
Enzymes, 81–82
    digestive, 114
    pancreatic, 114
    salivary gland, 81–82, 82
Esophageal sphincter
    lower, 41
Esophagitis, 11
Esophagus
    anatomy of, 41
Evidence

weighing, 72–73
Evidence-based medicine, 68–72
Exercise, 107, 121
Exercises
    group, 107
    Kegel, 108–109
    pelvic muscle, 108–109
    progressive muscle relaxation,
        120, 124–127
    strengthening, 107
    stretching, 107
Ex-Lax, 137
External sphincter, 86

F
Faltus-producing foods, 98–99
Family, 49–50
Fat absorption, 83–84
Fatigue, 8
Fatty foods
    emptying from stomach, 43
FDA. *See* Food and Drug
        Administration (FDA)
Fear
    gastric emptying, 44
Fecal softeners, 136
Fecal transplantation, 164–165
Fiber
    dietary, 86–93
        changing, 87
        increasing, 88–92
    products, 133–135
    soluble, 88
    supplements, 92–93
    types of, 87–88
First date diarrhea, 1–2
Flatulence, 33
    reducing, 98–99
Fletcher's Castoria, 137

Holtmann, Gerald, 49

Hormone
    abnormal release, 58–59

Hot peppermint teas, 144

Humor therapy, 121–122

Hydrochloric acid, 43, 83

Hydrogen, 100

Hypnosis, 131

Hypothesis, 58

Hysterectomy, 32

I

Iberis amara, 115

IBS. *See* Irritable bowel syndrome (IBS)

ICC. *See* Interstitial cells of Cajal (ICC)

IFFGD. *See* International Foundation for Functional Gastrointestinal Disorders (IFFGD)

Ileocecal valve, 85

Imagery, 122

Immune system, 107

Immunoglobulin G antibodies, 103

Imodium, 140–141, 150–151, 159

Imodium A-D, 140–141

Imodium Advanced, 140–141

Independent review board (IRB), 75

Indigestion, 33

Infection, 50–51

Inflammatory changes, 51

Information, 60

Inheritance, 49–50

Intelligence, 63

Internal anal sphincter, 86

International Foundation for Functional Gastrointestinal Disorders (IFFGD), 123–124, 124f, 167–168

Internet, 60, 69, 169–170

Interstitial cells of Cajal (ICC), 44

Intolerance
    foods, 101–104, 103f
        testing for, 104

IRB. *See* Independent review board (IRB)

Irrigation
    colonic, 105

Irritable bowel syndrome (IBS)
    cost of, 19–22
    defined, 3–5
    diagnosis, 25–38
    etiology, 46–49
    personal search to understand, 12–14
    prevalence of, 6f, 23–25
    symptoms of, 6–12, 25–33
    tests for, 25–33

Ispaghula, 133

J

Jesuits, 14

Journalizing, 123

Journals
    medical, 168–169
    research published in, 69

K

Kaopectate, 142

Kappa agonists, 165